Haemophilia in Aotearoa New Zealand
More Than A Bleeding Nuisance

Haemophilia in Aotearoa New Zealand provides a richly detailed analysis of the experience of the bleeding disorder of haemophilia based on long-term ethnographic research. The chapters consider experiences of diagnosis; how parents, children, and adults care and integrate medical routines into family life; the creation of a gendered haemophilia; the use and ethical dilemmas of new technologies for treatment, testing and reproduction; and how individuals and the haemophilia community experienced the infected blood tragedy and its aftermath, which included extended and ultimately successful political struggles with the neoliberalising state. The authors reveal a complex interplay of cultural values and present a close-up view of the effects of health system reforms on lives and communities. While the book focuses on the local biology of haemophilia in Aotearoa New Zealand, the analysis allows for comparison with haemophilia elsewhere and with other chronic and genetic conditions.

Julie Park is Professor Emerita of Anthropology at the University of Auckland, New Zealand.

Kathryn M. Scott works in social research and advocacy. She is an Honorary Research Fellow in Anthropology at the University of Auckland, New Zealand.

Deon York works in the health sector. He is currently President of the Haemophilia Foundation of New Zealand (HFNZ) and on the Board of Directors of the World Federation of Hemophilia (WFH).

Michael Carnahan has worked in health services management and is former President of the Haemophilia Foundation of New Zealand (HFNZ).

Routledge Studies in Health and Medical Anthropology

Haemophilia in Aotearoa New Zealand

More Than A Bleeding Nuisance

Julie Park, Kathryn M. Scott,
Deon York, and Michael Carnahan

Routledge
Taylor & Francis Group

LONDON AND NEW YORK

First published 2019
by Routledge
2 Park Square, Milton Park, Abingdon, Oxon OX14 4RN

and by Routledge
52 Vanderbilt Avenue, New York, NY 10017

First issued in paperback 2020

Routledge is an imprint of the Taylor & Francis Group, an informa business

British Library Cataloguing-in-Publication Data
A catalogue record for this book is available from the British Library

Library of Congress Cataloging-in-Publication Data
A catalog record has been requested for this book

ISBN 13: 978-0-367-66234-9 (pbk)
ISBN 13: 978-0-367-13444-0 (hbk)

Typeset in Sabon LT Std
by Cenveo® Publisher Services

To all people with haemophilia and those who care for them.

Contents

List of figures and tables

Figures

Table

List of boxes

Abbreviations

ACC	Accident Compensation Corporation (initially Commission), established in 1974
AIDS	Acquired immunodeficiency syndrome
AGM	Annual General Meeting
BTAC	Blood Transfusion Advisory Committee (NZ)
CDC	Centres for Disease Control (US)
CHE	Crown Health Enterprise: the name for erstwhile hospitals under the RHAs (New Zealand)
CSL	Commonwealth Serum Laboratories established 1916 by the Australian Government, which processed New Zealand blood. Established in 1991 as a public company and now named CSL Behring
CVS	Chorionic villus sampling: a prenatal testing method using the hair-like structures or villi
DHB	District Health Board: 21 (currently 20) of these were established in NZ in 2000 to fund and provide public health services
DNA	Deoxyribonucleic acid carries genetic instructions for growth and development, for functioning, and for reproduction
FVIII	Factor Eight: Haemophilia A
FIX	Factor Nine: Haemophilia B
GE or GM	Genetic engineering or Genetic modification
GP	General Practitioner: Family medicine doctor
HCV	Hepatitis C virus
HFNZ	Haemophilia Foundation of New Zealand (Inc)
HIV	Human immunodeficiency virus
IV	Intravenous
IVF	In vitro fertilisation: used in conjunction with PGD for haemophilia
NHMG	National Haemophilia Management Group, established 2006
NGO	Nongovernment Organisations

NZHS	New Zealand Haemophilia Society Inc (former name of HFNZ)
PCR	Polymerase chain reaction: a technique that allows small pieces of DNA to be replicated
PGD	Preimplantation genetic diagnosis of embryos
PHARMAC	Pharmaceutical Management Authority, established in June 1993
PHO	Primary Health Organisations
RHA	Regional Health Authority: four of these spanned NZ from 1993–97
RNA	RNA or ribonucleic acid is a molecule required to create proteins and is part of a qualitative blood test to determine the presence of hepatitis C in the bloodstream
TNV	The next virus - A reference to unknown viruses that may be transmitted by treatment products
WFH	World Federation of Hemophilia

Acknowledgments

Members of the haemophilia community have shared their stories and sometimes their lives with us in the hope that this research may help others. Our wish is that this book will fulfil this hope. We thank you all: people with haemophilia, clinical specialists, haemophilia nurses, outreach workers, council members, and staff of the Haemophilia Foundation and the many volunteers.

Anthropology colleagues: Christine Dureau, Ruth Fitzgerald, Judith Littleton, Maureen Molloy, Cris Shore, Samuel Taylor Alexander, Susanna Trnka, Catherine Trundle; graduate students in 'Reading Medical Anthropology' (2014): Natalie Daddy, Sarah Haggar, Lakna Jayasinghe, Julie Neville, Sally Raudon, Paul Robertson, Shirin Tuiti; Foundation officers: Richard Chambers, Chantel Lauzon; haemophilia specialists, Julia Phillips and B.J. Ramsay read and commented on earlier versions of individual chapters or the whole manuscript. We are extremely grateful to Laura McLauchlan and Sarah Haggar who brought their fresh eyes to different iterations of the whole manuscript. We acknowledge Elizabeth Berry and John Benseman who helped initiate this research. We thank you all and shoulder responsibility for the remaining errors and infelicities.

Tim Mackrell, Imaging Technologist, Anthropology, School of Social Science, created Figures 1.1, 1.3, 3.2, 4.4, and 5.1, and edited all the figures; Laura McLauchlan created Figures 4.1, 4.2, and 4.3, Edurne Scott Loinaz prepared Figures 6.1 and 6.2. Photo credits for Figures 2.1, and 4.4: Julie Park; Figure 3.1: Mike Carnahan; Figure 3.2: HFNZ. Kate Longmuir assisted with reference checking. Diane Lowther skilfully prepared the index.

Julie acknowledges her PhD students, Pauline Herbst and Kate Longmuir, whose conversations have helped clarify many ideas. She celebrates the continuing support of Judith Huntsman and thanks her coresearchers on other medical anthropological projects: Ruth Fitzgerald and Judith Littleton, and their forbearance as she worked on this one.

This research was supported financially by the Health Research Council of New Zealand, the Faculty of Arts and the Anthropology Department of the University of Auckland. Julie acknowledges the support of colleagues and her Department throughout the years of the project, and the Irish

Haemophilia Society, which allowed her to research in their archives in Dublin. Kathryn gratefully acknowledges her Manaaki Whenua Landcare Research Sustainable Settlements Scholarship and the University of Auckland Doctoral Scholarship, which supported the research on which Chapter 6 is based. Thanks to the *RAL* Editorial Board for permission to use material from *RAL* 5 and 8, and CEO of HFNZ, Richard Chambers, for items for Figure 3.2 and Box 7.1.

We are grateful for the Forewords by Jan-Willem André de la Porte and Elizabeth Berry. We thank the Haemophilia Foundation of New Zealand, which generously made its archives available and provided assistance throughout. The Foundation will receive all royalties from this publication.

Finally, we thank one another.

Foreword

Jan-Willem André de la Porte

The World Federation of Hemophilia (WFH), established in 1963, is an international not-for-profit with a growing global network of patient organizations, currently 140, and has official recognition from the World Health Organization.

The mission of the WFH is to improve and sustain care for people with inherited bleeding disorders all over the world. In achieving its goals, the WFH is faced with many contrasting realities and immense challenges to assist the almost 75 percent of people affected by a bleeding disorder with limited or no treatment.

Each local reality has its unique challenges. Have people been identified? Once they have been identified, what is the level of medical expertise and government support available to them? Are crucial therapies and infrastructure available in proximity that is practical for them? Alongside these challenges is the society and culture in which people affected by bleeding disorders are situated. Communities all over the world have both complementary and contrasting ideas about bleeding disorders, which are deeply connected to the culture and society of origin.

I was born in the Netherlands, and our family moved to South Africa where I was raised and educated. I have witnessed many changes to the treatment I receive, from 3 litres of plasma then, to 2.5ml of concentrate now, and ideas about what haemophilia is and what it means to live with it. On the vast African continent, specific cultural knowledges coexist with therapies used all over the world in areas fortunate enough to have access. Ideas about health and well-being are so engrained in societies, and understanding these is an important step to make improvements.

The Haemophilia Foundation of New Zealand (HFNZ) became an official member of the WFH from 1975, after a decade of association. Since 1958, when HFNZ was established, there have been significant changes in how haemophilia and related bleeding disorders have been treated locally. Changes in technology and how we view living with haemophilia have dramatically shifted.

Following many years of research, *Haemophilia in Aotearoa New Zealand: More than a Bleeding Nuisance* captures what it means to live with haemophilia and related bleeding disorders in New Zealand from the perspective of those who are the experts—the people and families affected every day. Equally important are the perspectives of the treaters and the system that supports people. In this community, voices of patients, family members, and treaters are given equal prominence—and this was the case long before it became fashionable.

What happens in New Zealand does not occur in a vacuum, with the New Zealand community being part of a global network of people who all face different challenges, but all advocate for appropriate infrastructure, training and technology to remain available to improve people's lives.

I congratulate the authors in documenting what it means to live in New Zealand with a bleeding disorder. This unique snapshot is as relevant locally as it is globally, and I hope it will inspire everyone to think more about how they can assist

Jan-Willem André de la Porte
Patron, World Federation of Hemophilia

Foreword

Dr Elizabeth Berry

This is a unique and fascinating social anthropology study of haemophilia in Aotearoa New Zealand that spans 20 years. It documents not only the history of haemophilia and its treatment through the lens of people with haemophilia and their families, but also provides considerable information on the impact of changes in the NZ health care system during that time and demonstrates the importance and effectiveness of political action.

My own association with the haemophilia community goes back 50 years—years of hope when comprehensive care and home therapy were introduced, despair and devastation due to HIV and hepatitis C viruses in the blood supply, then optimism as less risky recombinant products became available. Courage, determination, stoicism, and enthusiasm continue to shine through. In this study, I was intrigued to learn that not being able to play the national game of rugby, with its deeply ingrained symbolism of masculinity and mateship, continues to be such a source of sorrow for many of the boys and their fathers.

The Haemophilia Foundation of New Zealand (HFNZ) has been very active in providing support and education to families, particularly through family camps, and has also played a pivotal role in political lobbying for up-to-date therapy and recompense for viral infections. Both campaigns were eventually successful, as was the next one, which addressed inequity in care and, with HFNZ working closely with clinicians, resulted in the establishment of the centrally funded National Haemophilia Management Group. Today's child born with haemophilia can expect to have minimal joint damage and to live a normal lifespan, but issues such as management of inhibitors, concerns over testing carrier status, and decisions about pregnancy persist. HFNZ continues to be an active member of the WFH and most recently completed a successful twin programme with Cambodia.

With its many strands, this very readable book gives food for thought for anyone with an interest in haemophilia, anthropology, or the structure and politics of health and related services in New Zealand. It could even provide a template to study another genetic disorder. The authors should be heartily congratulated.

Elizabeth Berry, QSO, MD
Patron HFNZ; Former Director Auckland
Hospital Haemophilia Centre

1 A bleeding nuisance in Aotearoa New Zealand

The human experience of haemophilia: an introduction

Through our stories of the experience of haemophilia in Aotearoa New Zealand we explore key issues of our time. These include questions such as 'How should we respond to the new and developing issues associated with treatment of genetic disorders; issues such as gene therapy and selective reproductive technologies?' Some issues are situated at the level of the state, such as 'How should the government's health budget be allocated?', 'How should health services be organised to care for or cure those with expensive or rare disorders?', 'How can patient groups make a difference to health systems?', or 'What are the state's responsibilities to its citizens when things go badly wrong in its health provision?' Some are deeply personal: 'How and when do I tell my becoming-partner that I have a genetic condition, or hepatitis C?' or 'Should I have a baby, knowing that it may have a serious genetic condition?' Some questions are specific to Aotearoa New Zealand, such as 'What has rugby got to do with haemophilia?' and 'What does this genetic condition reveal about this society and culture?'

Haemophilia is widely understood in medical terms as a rare bleeding disorder resulting from genetic mutations that are passed down through generations. Progress in medical sciences means that haemophilia and its treatment are now well—but not completely—understood. But what is it like to live with a genetic bleeding disorder in which blood takes too long to clot? And what can research with people with haemophilia contribute to improved health services and understandings of local culture?

Discussions of and some answers to these questions emerge from this story of New Zealanders' lives, of who cares, of parents and children, of struggle, of community, of sex and gender, of citizen and State, of Māori and Pākehā. It is an uplifting story but it has its darker side. The people in this story are those with the genetic make-up that produces haemophilia, their families, their health professionals, and others involved. The story is based on two decades of anthropological engagement in the New Zealand haemophilia community and offers often unexpected views into life and cultural values. We analyse what certain key events and processes have meant to and for people with haemophilia. These include the changing context for health and health care provided by successive health 'reforms', the advent and aftermath of blood-borne viruses, the role of the state, the turn from dependence on voluntary blood donations to the use of international pharmaceuticals in haemophilia treatment, the increasing availability of genetic/reproductive technologies, and the emerging importance for the community of honouring the relationship between indigenous Māori and the Crown, initially established by the 1840 Treaty of Waitangi.

In this chapter, we introduce people with haemophilia as a diverse group within Aotearoa New Zealand and haemophilia as a diverse condition. To understand this diversity, we draw on and explain some medical anthropological theory. Our participatory research with people with haemophilia is described, along with the relevant biographical details of the authors. By being clear about what our studies are based on and the vantage points of the different authors we hope readers will be able to better judge our arguments and conclusions. We sketch in some of the characteristics of Aotearoa New Zealand society, the changing health systems, and the changing treatments for haemophilia and its complications, which all interact to shape how people with haemophilia live. The chapter ends with a preview of the book's chapters.

The label 'people with haemophilia' may promote the idea of a homogenous group with similar experiences, but we will show that while the life experiences of all members are shaped by what they have in common—haemophilia—these experiences differ. This is not just because people 'deal with it'[1] differently in the psychological sense, but because the year they were born, where they live and have lived, the type and severity of haemophilia they have, their gender, age, and social situation all interact to produce 'different' haemophilias. The aim, therefore, of this book is to trace how these dimensions coalesce in varied ways. We ask how the actions of people with haemophilia, individually and collectively, have been part of the process of creating different haemophilias as they negotiate the everyday of New Zealand society and make visible some of the taken-for-granted cultural, social, and political aspects of the society they, and we authors, share. Throughout, the theme of 'different haemophilias' permeates.

Our emphasis on haemophilia in New Zealand being a specific rather than a universal experience opens up the possibility for readers in other contexts to compare and contrast this story with their own experience or knowledge. It adds an ethnographically specific case study demonstrating that even a single gene condition like haemophilia is a social, cultural, economic, and political phenomenon. Readers in closely aligned nations, such as Australia, where members of haemophilia communities have long worked together with those from New Zealand, will find much that is familiar. Australian and New Zealand haemophilia specialists, for example, have coproduced a consensus statement on the challenges they see in haemophilia care and how to address them (Brown *et al.* 2015). Similarly, the national haemophilia organisations have had many exchanges and inter-actions. But each nation or state has its own health system (and reforms), and has charted alternate paths through the crises of infected blood and the challenges of new technologies. Readers in other nations, such as the Republic of Ireland, will be struck with the differences, as well as similar-ities, in the experiences of virus-infected blood, and readers everywhere will find some aspects of New Zealand's health services or culture curious.

People living with haemophilia in New Zealand are diverse: a cross-section numbering several hundred of the national population of around 4.7 million, selected not by a random survey but by the random generation and inheritance of genetic mutations. Biologically, haemophilia is diverse too, as the medically based explanations we introduce later in this chapter explain. Social, historical, and health service contexts have changed markedly over the last few decades and across the nation. Many people minimise haemophilia: as an elderly man we interviewed wryly observed, it's just 'a bleeding nuisance' (Park *et al.* 1995, 1). Parents school themselves and those around them to treat their son as 'a boy first and a haemophilia second', reminding themselves that he is 'the same little boy' after the diagnosis as he was before it, and not 'living' haemophilia. But for a minority, bad memories of their father's or other older relatives' suffering with haemophilia dominate. Their experience means that they see haemo-philia as so overwhelming that they take steps to avoid passing it into the next generation. As one woman who was undergoing assisted reproduction to avoid haemophilia said: 'From an early age I knew that I would not have a child with haemophilia' (Park and York 2008, 40).

Throughout the book, we often refer to 'the haemophilia community.' For many it is a face-to-face community as people come together for work-shops, camps, meetings, and conferences and, for almost all, it is also an imagined community that is often involved in mediated conversations and imaginatively shared experiences. What Anderson (1991 [1983]) suggested for the sense of belonging to a nation also has salience for this specific com-munity. Anderson posited that the realisation by individual readers that they share a daily reading of the same national newspaper was historically key to the imagined community of the nation. For the haemophilia commu-nity, the realisation by families that their frequent routines of intravenous transfusion of clotting factor are shared across the community provides a similar, but more embodied, sense of community. By community we do not suggest that it is always a unit, or unified, or that everyone within it has the same views. Rather, it is a series of interlocking networks that share con-nections—and not only to the condition of haemophilia. Shared struggles, shared experiences, shared conversations, mutual help, working and play-ing together, reading the haemophilia newsletter, *Bloodline*, and participat-ing in social media all create a biosocial community (Rabinow 1996; Rose and Novas 2005). The strength of feelings of membership in this commu-nity was vividly demonstrated at an AGM when hot debate erupted over the design of a new logo. The passionate but differentiated belonging to 'their' community was evinced by the emotion in the debate over this beloved community symbol (Cohen 1985).

In grappling with the diversity of haemophilia, we have been influenced by Lock's (2001) concept of 'local biologies' and Mol's (2002) discussion of difference, multiplicity, and unity in relation to arthrosclerosis. Consequently, we use these concepts to provide an overarching framework for our national study. Local biology takes us beyond the commonplace understanding that illness will be perceived differently in different times and places, to an analysis of how local historical, environmental, social, and cultural circumstances interacting with biology produce different bodily experiences and meanings of health and illness. For example, older people told us how 'before [blood clotting factor] concentrates' or 'before home treatment', they would not have dreamed of travelling overseas, going away for days on a yacht, or even going to a five-day music festival. Pain relief, which was such a vexed issue before effective treatment and brought with it great anxieties about addiction, is now less important for most, but not all, because adequate treatment is the best preventative for pain. With factor concentrates and the ability to treat oneself, haemophilia is now an appreciably different condition than it was three decades ago. It is different physically and different in the way it is imagined. People with it can now have different dreams. Different local biologies form over time and also over space. In Aotearoa New Zealand, we argue that the particular contemporary, local, social context with its cultural values, moral preoccupations, and political-economic structures, produces a local biology of haemophilia.

Mol's analysis differs from local biology, although she too is concerned with difference. Her study in the Netherlands demonstrated that arthrosclerosis was different depending on the vantage point of the person experiencing it. For an older person suffering from it, arthrosclerosis might be the inability to climb up the stairs, for a clinician supporting a person with it, it was the clinical signs, for a pathologist identifying it through the microscope it was the plaques on the blood vessels. Mol showed how the 'it' of arthrosclerosis was only brought into a single entity through much labour, especially bureaucratic labour, and there was contestation, for example, between the clinical and the pathologist's gaze, as to how that singular disease was constituted. Her work provides additional insights into difference, even within a certain local biology, and leads into the realm of studies of diagnosis (Jutel 2011). In our work on the variety of issues arising from our study of haemophilia, for example, gender, new technologies, or health advocacy, we have been influenced by these diverse theoretical perspectives, which we discuss in more detail in the relevant chapters.

We authors recognise that ethnographic research is a shared endeavour that results in the joint production of narratives. As researchers, we have offered respectful attention (Bourdieu *et al.* 1999, 607) to people living with haemophilia, and critical reflection on having haemophilia and working in the haemophilia community. Two of the authors have haemophilia themselves and both have been deeply involved in the Haemophilia Foundation of New Zealand (HFNZ). Three of the authors have backgrounds in anthropology and two were university-based anthropologists at the time of writing. Two have worked in the New Zealand health system, and one continues to do so. Our ethnographic research with and by people with haemophilia over a generation throughout New Zealand has yielded rich stories and experiences of what living with haemophilia means in these specific times and places. Through this work we (Julie and Kathryn, because Deon and Mike knew this all along) discovered complexity and simplicity: complexity entailing the need to write about different haemophilias and simplicity expressed in our participants' hopes, such as, 'I want to live a normal life' or 'I just want to know I will be looked after when I get sick'. Our accounts try to represent complexity and simplicity, diversity and commonality, and to show how these dimensions of the experiences of our participants are created. The experiences are multiplex, but share a medical diagnosis of haemophilia.

Biogenetic haemophilias

In medical terms, haemophilia refers to coagulation disorders caused by mutations on specific genes located on the X chromosome. Haemophilia also occurs in other species, dogs for example, and appears to occur in all human populations. The most common type of haemophilia, haemophilia A, a deficiency in clotting factor VIII (eight), has a reported incidence of approximately one in every 10,000 births in the human species. Haemophilia B, factor IX (nine) deficiency, is less common at 1 in 50,000 births (Pruthi 2005; WFH 2012). About 30 per cent of haemophilia is 'sporadic', that is, a result of a new mutation in that individual or their mother. It subsequently will be inherited in the usual way. While there are commonly occurring mutations, less common ones have led to difficulties in diagnosis for some people. The inheritance pattern of these recessive X-linked conditions means that, at a population level, for every man with haemophilia, three women will be carriers of the mutation. All the daughters of men with haemophilia inherit their father's mutation but none of the sons do. The children of women with the mutation each have a 50-50 chance of inheriting it (see Figure 1.1). Some women carriers also experience bleeding problems and have clotting factor levels low enough to give them haemophilia (WFH 2012). People with haemophilia have much less clotting factor than normal in their blood; hence bleeding can arise spontaneously or from trauma and the bleed is very slow to stop.

In its mildest forms, sometimes divided into two categories of very mild and mild (between 5 per cent and 40 per cent of normal clotting factor), haemophilia may cause few problems in daily life, and may be an issue only if an accident occurs or if surgery is contemplated. Moderate

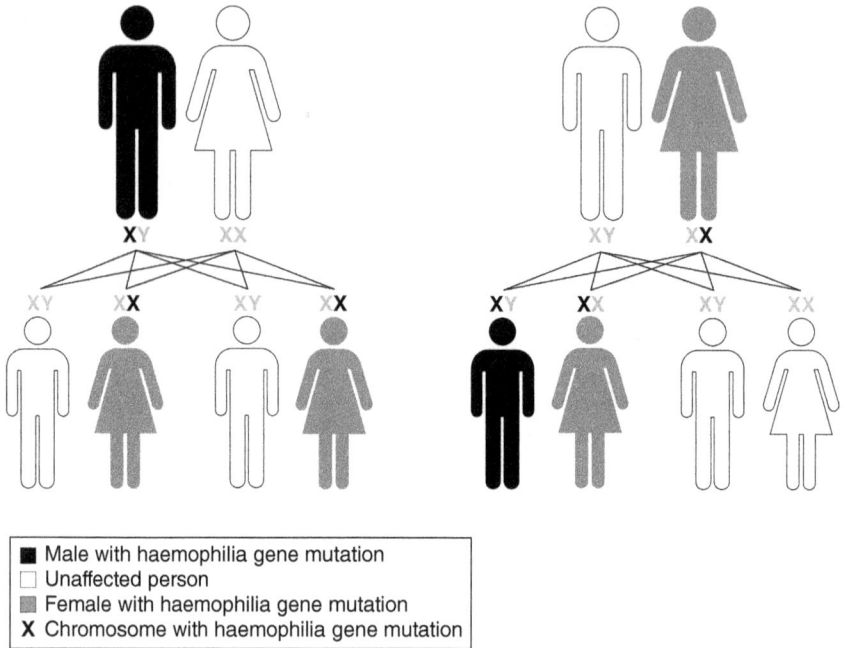

Male with haemophilia gene mutation
Unaffected person
Female with haemophilia gene mutation
X Chromosome with haemophilia gene mutation

Figure 1.1 Inheritance of haemophilia.

(between 1 to 5 per cent) or severe (less than 1 per cent of normal clotting factor) haemophilia can cause major disruptions to daily living, severe health problems, consequent difficulties in education, employment, and early death. However, individuals often have varying patterns of bleeds even with the same clotting factor levels. Severe haemophilia affects mainly males (Roberts and Jones 1990) although very occasionally women may also have less than 1 per cent of normal levels of clotting factor. Without clotting factor replacement treatment, bleeding for people with severe and some with moderate haemophilia may start spontaneously at any time, or as a result of even minor knocks or twists. Repeated bleeds into joints, called 'target joints', and muscles will cause long-term damage, intense pain and, eventually, permanent mobility problems; bleeds into organs, and especially into the central nervous system, may be life threatening.

In New Zealand and in many of the more affluent countries, treatment by intravenous infusion of replacement clotting factor has been available for decades for people with haemophilia (Ockelford *et al.* 1989). This treatment allows them to take part in most everyday activities, helps reduce the effects of trauma, and means children will have average life expectancy. However, in less-developed countries, treatment is usually available only to the privileged few. The World Federation of Hemophilia estimates that 75 per cent of the world receives little or inadequate treatment and has a programme to ameliorate this (WFH 2015). A major complication of treatment is the development of antibodies, known as inhibitors, that reduce the effectiveness of treatment in up to 20 per cent of people treated.

The historical context of haemophilia in Aotearoa New Zealand

What has happened over time and space is important in creating different haemophilias. Over the last half-century, similar to most of the developed world, New Zealanders with haemophilia have experienced great improvements in treatment and services allowing many to lead what they consider 'a pretty normal life' and to think of haemophilia as 'not serious really' or 'not a life-threatening disease'. But due to blood-borne infections, this life- and freedom-giving treatment has also been life-taking and health-limiting. Some have died, others have become very sick, and a number may become sick in the future. Our study documents the political and personal consequences of HIV and hepatitis C in New Zealand's blood supply, and especially the struggle for a safe blood supply and advocacy for redress. This aspect of our work adds to the array of accounts of 'bad blood' in haemophilia communities around the world and to studies of biosocial citizenship (Kirp 1999; Resnik 1999; Taylor and Power 2011).

Health and illness are processes that people negotiate in particular cultural, historical and political settings. The struggles for recognition and redress for HIV and hepatitis C were driven by strong New Zealand cultural values of egalitarianism and the right to a 'fair go', meaning that individuals and groups should have equal rights to justice and fair recompense. The historian Fischer's (2012) detailed study of key moral values in the United States and New Zealand suggests that, although both countries share values, the emphases are different. Fairness triumphs in New Zealand; freedom in the United States. Fairness can have various meanings and may relate to individuals or society, but the concept of equity or 'a fair go' has had a long history here and has accumulated a well-developed language (Belich and Wevers 2008). We suggest that much of New Zealand's social provision, including its health system, is governed and received in the context of this value, even in the midst of neoliberal reforms. As Reid (2015) points out in the context of health, equity or fairness do not equate to sameness. What is at stake is equity in provision and outcome.

The experience of four sets of health reforms in New Zealand over a period of two decades has created different experiences of haemophilia, at times increasing inequity in service provision, at other times enhancing access and quality of care. Later in this chapter, we chart these changes as they are relevant to people with haemophilia. As a condition that requires a wide range of services for comprehensive treatment, haemophilia presents something of a test case for health reforms, including funding structures, health service provision and associated welfare services. The New Zealand health restructurings have attracted interest at home and abroad from scholars, politicians, and health experts (Ashton 2005; Gauld 2009; Laugesen and Gauld 2012; Okma and Crivelli 2010). Our study documents their complex effects on real people, 'the inscribing of historical time onto flesh' (Fassin 2007, xv), which Fassin maintains is one of the tasks of anthropology. We show too that people with haemophilia also produce effects on New Zealand health systems.

Living with haemophilia

For every man or woman who carries a gene mutation for haemophilia several others are living with haemophilia. These include family members, friends, partners, teachers, employers and those caregivers in health and social services who, over the years and sometimes generations, develop close links with people with haemophilia. Estimates vary for the number of people who have haemophilia in New Zealand. In March 1994, 520 people were listed as having haemophilia in the Haemophilia Society of New Zealand's 'Standards of Care' (HFNZ Archives), but at the end of 1994, 583 men and 40 women 'expressed carriers' were noted on an informal national haemophilia register for New Zealand (Park *et al.* 1995, 217). This number included over 100 people with very mild haemophilia. A total of 433 men and 224 women carriers was cited shortly after by the Joint RHA Project (1996, 22–3) (see Table 1.1). The differences in these figures are mainly related to the enumeration of those in the mild and very mild categories, a difference in the 'cut-off' between severe and moderate (2% vs 1%), and the inclusion of women carriers. Haemophilia is a continuum and establishing boundaries at the very mild end is problematic. Given the

Table 1.1 Estimated numbers of people with haemophilia: 1994[1]–6[2] and 2015[3]

Type	Severity	1994	1996	2015
Factor VIII	Severe	103/86	118	135
Haemophilia A	Moderate	29/49	36	62
	Mild	238/282	189	280
	Very mild	69/0		
		439/417	**343**	**477**
Factor IX	Severe	21/15	29	32
Haemophilia B	Moderate	22/29	25	50
	Mild	28/16	26	36
	Very mild	10/0		
		81/60	**80**	**118**
Total		**520/477**	**423**	**595**

Sources:

1) New Zealand Haemophilia Society Inc. (March 1994) *Standards of Care.*/National Haemophilia Register 1994, Haemophilia Foundation of New Zealand Archives.
2) Joint Regional Health Authority Project Team. 1996, 22-23.
3) Records collated by Deon York and BJ Ramsay, 16 Oct, 2015.

number (350) of our questionnaires sent out by the various treatment centres to people with haemophilia who were patients or parents of patients,
a figure of somewhat over 350 for people who were actually being treated
for haemophilia seems to be realistic for 1994. This number, 350, would
underestimate those with mild haemophilia who did not require treatment.
The clinicians also may have not sent questionnaires to some patients. By
2014 the National Haemophilia Management Group maintained a national
register (Julia Phillips, *pers. comm.* January 1, 2015), and the estimated
number of people with haemophilia, according to HFNZ was at least 430
(HFNZ 2016a) with 182 people with haemophilia having been born since
1989 (Chantel Lauzon *pers. comm.* March 2014). In October 2015, returns
from all centres treating people with haemophilia were collated by Deon
York and B.J. Ramsay (Clinical Nurse Specialist, Haemophilia Centre,
Wellington). A figure of 477 with haemophilia A and 118 with haemophilia B,
totalling 595 was reached, with a note that the mild category is the least
reliable. A figure of around 600 seems a reasonable current estimate for
people who have received a diagnosis of haemophilia.

Treatment for haemophilia

Treatment is available in the form of transfusions of the missing clotting factors, either derived from plasma or synthetically manufactured
(Peyvandi and Garagiola 2015; Rosendaal *et al.* 1991). By 2014, those people who remained on plasma-derived treatment comprised those for whom
there was a clinical reason not to change or those who had chosen not to
use recombinant products because they were satisfied with the quality and
safety of the blood products; often patients opted not to change because
they feared a change could trigger inhibitors. Otherwise, New Zealanders
use synthetic recombinant products. For younger New Zealanders with
severe and sometimes moderate haemophilia, prophylactic infusion of clotting factor replacement to prevent bleeds is used; that is, regular treatments
several times a week using the same products as for on-demand treatment,
which treats after a bleed has begun. Older folk often treat on demand as
usually they experience fewer bleeds. Whether a person has haemophilia
A or B determines what specific clotting factor product will be suitable
to assist blood clotting and bring bleeding to a halt or prevent it starting. Depending on the type and severity of haemophilia and little understood personal factors, between one and 20 per cent of people on treatment
develop inhibitors, which are antibodies that destroy factor VIII or IX,
causing great difficulties in treatment (HFNZ 2016b). There are many further intricacies of haemophilia that recourse to a haematology text or haemophilia Internet sites will describe.

Treatment has progressed over recent decades as we detail in chapter 4,
but many older people with haemophilia suffer from the long-term effects
of no or inadequate treatment in earlier years, particularly joint damage,

and many of their age cohorts died untimely deaths due to the condition. Although haemophilia treatment is effective, there is no cure as yet and at present, a child born with the disorder will have it for the rest of his or her life. Haemophilia is one of the more expensive conditions to treat. About $25 million per year is spent on treatment products in New Zealand (PHARMAC 2015). Hope for the future involves the use and refinement of recombinant clotting factors to create products that are easier to administer and require much less-frequent treatment. Gene therapy also holds promise.

Comprehensive treatment does not stop with clotting factor replacement and haematology but may include physiotherapy, specialised dentistry, orthopaedic work and orthotics, gynaecology, specialist obstetrics, and paediatric services. Various counselling and social work services may also be required. Some younger patients may require educational help, and older ones some assistance with employment or income maintenance. Genetic testing services and genetic counselling are also used by some people. In addition, to keep healthy and well despite haemophilia requires good primary care and systems of referral. Some people find complementary medicine helpful in relieving some of the symptoms of haemophilia, such as painful joints. As a result of blood-borne infections, many people with haemophilia born before 1993 also suffered from one or more infectious diseases that needed to be treated by gastroenterologists and other infectious disease specialists. This one condition therefore requires a very comprehensive system of care. And people with haemophilia are subject to the same other illnesses as others in the community and any surgical intervention, no matter how minor, requires extra precautions. Our long-term research with people with haemophilia in the context of continuing health reforms provided a window into the lived effects of health-system restructuring and the collective attempts of people with haemophilia to create a satisfactory health system for themselves and others.

The view from now

As we write in the second decade of the twenty-first century, life with haemophilia now looks very different from even 30 years ago. Children can expect to attend school regularly and experience little pain, although pain cannot be avoided entirely. Despite recent research indicating that even with excellent prophylaxis microbleeds still cause long-term damage (Clement 2014), as youngsters age, their joints will not deteriorate like those of current elders. As young adults, a greater range of tertiary education and employment options will be available for them. If they wish, they can confidently enter long-term relationships, have children, and expect to live long enough to see their grandchildren with a life expectancy close to normal. Many formerly impossible leisure pursuits and voluntary activities are available to them. Treatments are still necessary, some limitations on physical activities remain, and sometimes extra caution is required with everyday tasks, such as using a screwdriver. Holidays and other travel need careful planning because treatment paraphernalia and doctors' letters have to be packed. Dental and medical procedures also need extra planning, and women with haemophilia may need extra help with menstruation and childbirth. But with good treatment, the goal of living 'a normal life' as a New Zealander is attainable.

Just as the experience of haemophilia has changed over time, so too have our research studies. The studies evolved to respond to the then current foci of the haemophilia community. Initially, this was to establish basic information about people with haemophilia, the standards of care they experienced, and what changes would be beneficial. Next, the issue of hepatitis C was at the forefront. By the final phase our foci included the government's response to the hepatitis C issue through its Treatment and Welfare Package, the creation of the National Haemophilia Management Group (NHMG), and the community's response to new technologies of treatment and new reproductive options. It is to the details of these studies that we now turn.

The 'Bleeding nuisance' studies

Beginning the research

In 1993, John Benseman, a social researcher and educationalist who has a son with haemophilia, was a member of the committee of the (then) New Zealand Haemophilia Society (NZHS, now HFNZ). As a social researcher with a particular interest in education, he was fascinated by the stories of his fellow committee members and people attending NZHS family camps. Listening to parents' stories about how they coped with ongoing stress and occasional crises led him to discuss such experiences with numerous people, including some of the older members. He realised that things were changing fast for people with haemophilia and almost no social research into the haemophilia community in New Zealand had been carried out. During these talks, John was encouraged to form a suitable research team and put together a grant application for funding, and to seek formal approval and cooperation from the Committee of NZHS. He approached Julie Park, a fellow researcher, newly appointed to a lectureship in the Department of Anthropology at the University of Auckland, to work with him. Julie's interest was piqued and she asked a recent Masters graduate in social anthropology, Kathryn Scott, to help. These three and Elizabeth Berry, then a consultant haematologist with particular responsibility for haemophilia care, formed the original research team for the 1994–5 study. Elizabeth's participation was crucial. Not only did she provide a respected bridge to generations of people with haemophilia, but she introduced Kathryn and Julie to other haematologists and specialists, and patiently discussed the complications of haemophilia with us. While formulating the proposal, our research group had discussions with NZHS committee members to strengthen our partnership approach. The proposal attracted 'small grant' funding ($50,000) from the Health Research Council of New Zealand, approval from the national ethics committee, and formally began in 1994.

The study was anthropological in its conception and involved documenting the everyday lives of people with haemophilia, seeking their perspectives on all aspects of their lives. The study also analysed the effects of changes in the treatment of haemophilia and the organisation of haemophilia and other government services in recent years. The continuing effects of past contamination of clotting factor concentrates constituted an important part of the study as did the related roles of people with haemophilia and their health professionals in support and advocacy. Carrying out this study in New Zealand where the population is small enough to enable a nationwide study provided methodological advantages and the opportunity to use a range of research methods.

Research design

Field research for the initial study began in June 1994. The final report was completed 18 months later (Park *et al.* 1995). The research philosophy underlying the project was one of partnership (Park 1992). The relationships established early in the research with members of the NZHS (now HFNZ) were maintained throughout the project including the reporting process. Similarly, through Elizabeth Berry, we had a relationship with several haematologists, who were also participants in the research, and other key people as we worked toward the recommendations for action that came out of the study.

The theoretical framework which we found most satisfactory and illuminating at this time was that of 'culture and political economy', which holds a tension between interpretative anthropology and political economy. This framework encourages us to imagine culture as contested and informed by difference, and to envisage power in terms that owe something to Foucault and to feminist analysis, as both productive and located at all levels, in all institutions and relationships (di Leonardo 1991, 27; Farmer 1992).

In developing our project design we wanted to highlight the day-to-day and lifelong experience of people with haemophilia and those close to them. This included an emphasis on family relationships and parenting, schooling, obtaining work, pursuing leisure activities, access to care, advice relating to haemophilia, and so on. However, we also wanted to research the history of people with haemophilia and their families as a political action group in the health field as well as the social, political and economic context of prevention and treatment of haemophilia and associated conditions.

Our approach therefore needed to be broad-ranging and multilevel. We adopted a multimethod approach, which generated both qualitative and quantitative data. Qualitative information was the main focus of the study and we compared information derived from various sources. As perceptive writers on research methods have long known (e.g., Hammersley and Atkinson 1983, 198–200), data from one source cannot be used as a simple check on data from another source. However, the exploration of interesting discrepancies can lead to more insightful research questions, better techniques, and more valid findings. Validity checks were provided by discussion between the researchers and between researchers and key persons. Adopting the 'funnel' strategy, initially described by Agar (1980, 9), we moved progressively from a broader to a narrower focus; thus the generalisability of our findings from the narrow end—interviews and participant observation—was considered in light of the findings at the broad end—the questionnaire.

Research methods 1994–5

In our initial study we collected statistical data from existing statistics of NZHS, the New Zealand Society for Haematology, and documentary and statistical data from the NZHS archive. We reviewed the international literature for social research relating to haemophilia or other conditions that were similar in some respects, and for research relating to the likely themes of our study. We conducted key person interviews with members of NZHS, haematologists, and relevant health service personnel and arranged focus groups with people with haemophilia and those who supported them to help develop a questionnaire to be used with the known national population. These focus groups provided important research insights, such as the importance of hepatitis C in the community. With the help of the seven Haemophilia Treatment Centres and NZHS, we invited people with haemophilia to take part in our study. In the days before Internet and cell phones, this invitation was via mail. We estimate that approximately 350 invitations were issued. Two hundred people replied, again by mail, wanting to take part. We wrote back, enclosing their questionnaire, a pen, and a tea bag, asking them to complete a comprehensive questionnaire, which included both quantitative and open-ended questions (see Figure 1.2). We received 193 completed questionnaires. Once the questionnaires were analysed, we interviewed in person approximately 80 people chosen to be a cross-section of questionnaire respondents, and, where possible, their families or significant others. This involved thousands of kilometres of driving. Throughout the research period, we participated in and observed various group situations where people with haemophilia came together, such as at meetings, camps, and celebrations. Once we had completed our draft report, we conferred with approximately 30 key persons, including through a lengthy workshop, by phone, and by mail before writing the recommendations.

Shortly after the 1994–5 phase was completed, a Masters student in Anthropology, Belinda Strookappe, joined the study to further explore the views and experiences of women carriers of haemophilia in relation

Living with Haemophilia in Aotearoa/New Zealand

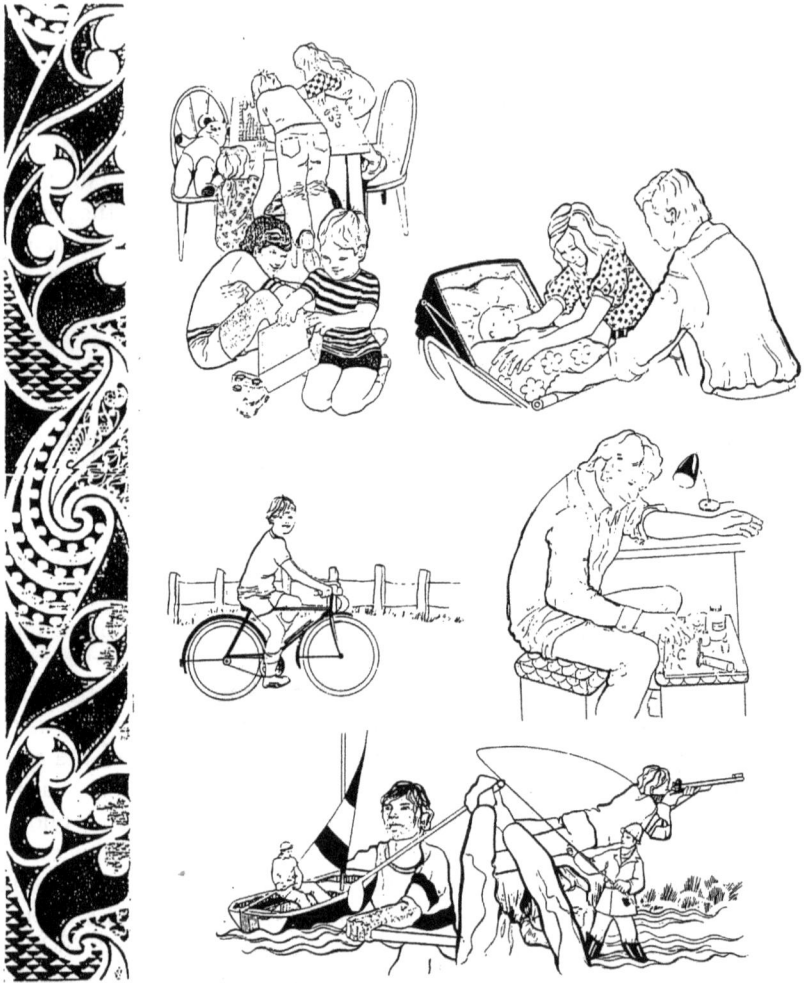

All information given will remain anonymous and totally confidential.

Please feel free to make comments in the margins.

Figure 1.2 Original questionnaire, 1994.

to having children. Belinda carried out nine more interviews with women in the Auckland region focussed on this topic (Park and Strookappe 1996; Strookappe 1996).

Participation initiated in 1994 continued throughout the two decades of involvement, in between the times spent doing interviews, questionnaires, or other specific research. Consequently, when we contacted a subset of our original participants in 1999 to update our study, we were still familiar to almost all of them.

Update studies

In 1999, we (Kathryn and Julie) undertook a small follow-up study using phone interviews, as neither time nor resources permitted us to travel. In this study, we reinterviewed people who were willing using sections of our original interview outline, updated as necessary, leaving the conversation open-ended. We chose a cross-section of those who had completed questionnaires in 1994–5 and concentrated on two areas: the experience of hepatitis C for those for whom this was relevant, and for everyone, general issues of daily living. Thirty people participated and half of them had direct experience with hepatitis C.

In 2003, Julie spent a few weeks of her sabbatical leave in Dublin reviewing some of the extensive materials in the archives of the Irish Haemophilia Society relating to their struggles with HIV and hepatitis C and talking with staff about the process and outcomes as a comparison with the New Zealand experience. In 2005–6, Deon York, a recent anthropology graduate and member of HFNZ, and Julie planned another update study, this time focussing on the social ecology of new therapies and technologies. Invitations to participate were issued through HFNZ. This study, too, was done with few resources, but included face-to-face (again Julie covered about 3,000 km interviewing in the North and South Islands) and phone interviews around four main areas: hepatitis C and new treatments available, new reproductive technologies, new treatments including gene therapy, and issues of daily living. Because of individual circumstances, each interview was unique although based around common topics. The 37 participants, interviewed in 33 sessions, included approximately half who had participated in earlier studies and half who were new to this research.

Participant observation at New Zealand Haemophilia Society and Foundation events was an important component of both update studies, as it had been in the initial study, our fieldnotes, and the minutes and documents from these gatherings: AGMs, planning meetings, camps, educational sessions, and celebrations, formed part of our research material. Interviews for both update studies were transcribed verbatim by the researchers and analysed following the same process of careful reading, definition of themes and cross-checking between researchers used in the initial study. Successive versions of the QSL software for qualitative analysis, up to N6 by the 2006 analysis, allowed for sophisticated exploration of our texts. All of this material, analysed in terms of the research questions and emerging themes, provided the basis for the report by Park and York (2008), academic articles, and conference presentations. The Faculty of Arts and the Department of Anthropology of the University of Auckland provided the small grants for both these updates.

Reflections on research

Anthropology at home is variously conceived. By most definitions this work would qualify. We researchers worked in our own country, in the same language group, and the participants share general understandings of social life as the researchers and authors (Strathern 1987). The research teams and the authors include people with and without haemophilia and move easily in the haemophilia community and in the wider society. The downside of this is overfamiliarity and taking-for-granted what should be questioned and further explored (Dyck 2000). For example, the roles of parent and patient expert (Trnka and McLauchlan 2012), the assumptions of fairness (Belich and Wevers 2008; Fischer 2012), and, as products of a welfare state, the 'of course' assumption that haemophilia care must come out of the public purse.

Anthropology at home often entails advocacy or engagement in political processes. This is true of this project both within HFNZ and on its behalf. For example, our initial study provided useful information on regional disparities in treatment to assist advocacy for national Standards of Haemophilia care (Park, Scott, and Benseman 1999). We attempted to share our findings widely with nonspecialists (Scott 1997). Our research also contributed the experiences of people with haemophilia and hepatitis C to an analysis of structural changes required in the blood service (Howden-Chapman *et al.* 1996) and was used by the Joint Regional Health Authority Project team on the purchasing and provision of haemophilia services (1996). Our, especially Carnahan's (2013) and Scott's (2013), analyses of the political processes leading to the resolution of the hepatitis C debacle and the institution of a National Haemophilia Management Committee have demonstrated how the actions of community groups can influence government policy. Inside the haemophilia community, our research indicated that there were areas of unmet need relating, for example, to women in the community, and to Māori. Our later studies made available the range of views and values on assisted reproduction within the community and contributed to more open discussions on this sensitive topic (Park and York 2008). These research opportunities to analyse aspects of Aotearoa New Zealand society through a haemophilia lens, and to consider some of the more universal challenges of our time, such as new technologies, the provision of effective health services, and community empowerment, have informed this book.

Two authors, Mike and Deon, are active members of the haemophilia community and have been on its council. Both have participated internationally, have been presidents of HFNZ, and research participants. Deon's term as president coincided with the preparation of this book. These involvements predated and will continue beyond our research. Julie and Kathryn's roles are as researchers and supporters of the haemophilia community.

Transformations in society and in health services

During the life of our research, New Zealand has been undergoing a remarkable transformation. Called 'the New Zealand experiment' by Kelsey (1997), and often dated to 1984, the change has been from a welfare state in which citizenship, participation, and belonging for all citizens was the goal (Royal Commission on Social Policy 1988), to a neoliberalised 'workfare' contracting state in which the ability to work underpins citizenship (Humpage 2015; McClure 1998, 232–4; McKenzie 1997). This has been accompanied by the marketisation of domains such as education and health, and shifting ideas of citizenship. Some changes in citizenship relate to the neoliberal active, self-responsible citizen, but others have to do with changing ideas of the nation, especially in relation to the Treaty of Waitangi, and Aotearoa New Zealand's place in the world.

The Treaty is regarded as the founding document of New Zealand, signed between Māori Chiefs and the representatives of Queen Victoria in 1840 at Waitangi and subsequently in various locations around Aotearoa New Zealand. The Treaty sets out the relationships between Māori and the Crown and is taken as the grounds on which non-Māori may settle in New Zealand. Fischer (2012, 295) suggests that this agreement was evidence of some common ground regarding fairness held by Māori and Pākehā at the time. Widely disregarded during much of the remainder of the nineteenth and the first three-quarters of the twentieth century by the Crown and the settler population, the Treaty was never forgotten by Māori. Effective activism led to the Treaty of Waitangi Act in 1975 and especially the 1985 Amendment. Under this act, groupings of Māori (usually iwi, 'tribes') and the Crown have been able to conduct research on the effects of colonisation and bring historical and contemporary claims and cases for apology and redress to the Waitangi Tribunal, which makes recommendations to the Crown. It seems likely that all major claims that are not yet settled will be settled in the next few years. This is a transformative process for Māori (15 per cent of the population) and for the nation as a whole, as iwi at long last recover mana, some of their economic base, and initiate social, environmental, and economic programmes. Māori institutions that have undergone transformation since European settlement have had a particularly intensive period of change as a result of the requirements of claims and settlement processes (Ballara 1998; Bell *et al.* 2017; Kawharu 2013).

During this neoliberalising period, New Zealand became more unequal, as measured by the Gini coefficient (OECD 2014; Rashbrooke 2013, 27). Increasing inequality has had complex effects on population health disparities, adversely impacting Māori and Pacific peoples, especially before the year 2000 (Woodward and Blakely 2014, 214–5). Rising house prices, especially in Auckland and other centres, have greatly outstripped rises in wages. The dream of a home of one's own, once a fundamental tenet of the good life for New Zealanders, is now more of a mirage for many, while more fortunate others benefit from the appreciation of property values. Renters do not have the protections found in many other nations and homelessness is an issue. Housing inequality, although not new, has become particularly acute in recent years (Howden-Chapman, Bierre, and Cunningham 2013). Wealth too has been increasingly concentrated in the hands of the few, with half the wealth being concentrated in the hands of just 10 per cent of the population by 2006 (Cheung 2007, 8). Despite these changes toward increased inequity, as Fischer (2012) points out, the rhetorical value of the concept of fairness has not diminished, and neoliberal repertoires are interwoven with values of participation and community, even among 'the children of Rogernomics' (i.e. of neoliberal policies) (Nairn, Higgins, and Sligo 2012).

Fairness was the reason why a 'first-past-the-post' system of electing representatives to the unicameral government was replaced by mixed-member proportional voting. Implemented in 1996, having been approved by a referendum in 1993, this has led to coalition governments and a more diverse set of representatives in parliament, somewhat more in tune with the increasingly diverse population. Of the population of roughly 4.5 million in 2015, people grouped into the 'Asian' category comprised 11.8 per cent of the population, while those grouped into 'Pacific' comprised 7.4 per cent (Statistics New Zealand 2015). 'Māori' were 14.9 per cent of the population, 'European' were 74 per cent and about three per cent were 'Other'. The numbers total more than 100 per cent because people choosing more than one ethnicity are represented in multiple categories. Recognition of increasing ethnic and cultural diversity and the diverse interests and needs of groupings based in gender and sexuality, age, disabilities, religion, and so on has been a feature of recent decades, expressed in such formal institutions as same-sex marriage (2013), building codes that mandate accessibility (Building Act 2004), the New Zealand Bill of Rights Acts (1990) and Human Rights Act (1993), and the adoption of New Zealand Sign Language in 2006 as the third official language with English and Māori. Although the outcomes of this formal recognition are far from perfect, the trend toward greater diversity and greater political recognition of diversity is incontrovertible.

Like Britain, New Zealand is a parliamentary democracy and constitutional monarchy. It has an 'unwritten' constitution in the sense that it is dispersed over many pieces of legislation. Unlike Britain, it has only a single House of Parliament, after a failed experiment in the nineteenth century with an upper and lower house and provinces. The Queen is the head of state, represented by a Governor General, who in recent years has been a New Zealander. As a former colony, dominion and now a nation, which is part of the commonwealth, New Zealand's ties with Britain go deep. For a long period, it prided itself as being a better Britain of the South Seas (Belich 2001) and a supplier of quality food to British people. But Britain's entry into the European community, the loss of special access to British markets, and other world events attenuated that tie to the point where New Zealand politicians in recent years frequently speak about New Zealand as an Asia Pacific nation (Haworth 1994; Lynch 2015). Brexit, the British vote to leave the EU in July 2016, seems unlikely to reverse this trend.

Values that underpin life in New Zealand, such as 'a fair go' are still invoked, are part of national ideology and enshrined in the Bill of Rights, enacted in 1990. For example, Section 25 provides for the right to a 'fair' hearing in criminal proceedings, and Section 27 invokes the principles of 'natural justice', which the architect of the Bill of Rights, Sir Geoffrey Palmer, explained was interchangeable with the concept of 'fairness' (Fischer 2012, 465). Socially liberal policies such as gay marriage have been enacted at the same time as economically regressive policies, such as stringent work-testing requirements for beneficiaries, increases in the Goods and Services Tax but no general capital gains tax. National-led governments' reforms to make a 'fairer' system of health care transformed the concept to equate to the 'level playing field' in a free market, rather than equitable access to resources. The 1991 health reforms, for example, introduced a requirement for fairness, which in this case referred to the ability of health consumers to choose between competitively funded health providers (Prince, Kearns, and Craig 2006). Yet, for those promoting health, fairness is much more fundamental and is about striving to reduce inequalities in health (Signal and Ratima 2015). Throughout this whole period, progressive settlements of Treaty of Waitangi claims have restored mana to many iwi, and provided the potential for economic, cultural and social recovery. It is this contradictory social and cultural landscape that provides the backdrop for changes in the health sector.

Health sector changes

Along with other branches of the public service, the health sector has been radically restructured as tensions between a social welfare foundation wrestled with privatisation, deregulation, cost containment in government spending, and other features of neoliberalism. People with haemophilia in New Zealand are intimately connected with publicly provided health services. Changes in the way that services are provided and in the services themselves create different haemophilias over time. The experiences of people living with haemophilia throughout the radical changes in health policy, structures, and care provide an opportunity to understand the meaning and effects of health service changes and other social policy changes for people in the community. Therefore, we ask how these reforms and their intended and unintended consequences were experienced by people with haemophilia. How did they change local biologies of haemophilia?

During the 1980s a series of escalating tensions in the public sector in general and specifically in health gave rise to a cascade of restructuring. These tensions revolved around attempts to curb escalating costs, to increase fairness of provision across the country, to balance power struggles between clinical services and community health, and to implement competition and market models instead of government paying for and providing services centrally.

Until the 1980s, the health sector was fragmented (Barnett and Barnett 2008) with a national Department of Health that had regional offices, many elected hospital boards, and private medical practitioners who delivered heavily subsidised primary care. Publicly funded District and Public Health nurses worked in the community. Multiple reviews of the health sector from the mid-1970s until the late-1980s declared that something had to be done to rationalise health care systems (Gibbs, Fraser, and Scott 1988). Between 1980 and 1990 something was done: Area Health Boards that integrated both hospital and public health services were formed, sometimes voluntarily, sometimes not. These elected boards were initiated in 1983 and numbered 14 by 1989. They operated within a regime of population-based funding and in accordance with national health goals. However, pressure on the public purse was not decreased, hospital waiting lists grew, and no marked improvement in equity of provision resulted. Nor did this change affect primary care.

Area Health Boards did not have the opportunity to prove their worth or otherwise because they were replaced by a markedly different system, announced in 1991 and fully implemented by 1993 (Blank 1994). This was the system newly in place when we began our research. This system created four Regional Health Authorities (RHAs) that purchased health services from public, private, and community providers, according to a funding formula that acknowledged areas of high population growth (see Figure 1.3). Public hospitals were renamed Crown Health Enterprises, and as their name suggests, they were corporatised, with directors appointed by government. RHAs also had government-appointed directors. This was the height of the market model that exacerbated tensions between managers and clinicians and further polarised their understandings of their roles (Fitzgerald 2004). However, the purchaser-provider split created opportunities for a range of different providers. These included community trusts, Māori providers, Pasifika providers, and organisations of general practitioners, such as Independent Practitioners Associations (IPAs), which contracted with RHAs. Keeping abreast of the new acronyms, let alone the new structures and arrangements, was a challenge. Some national-level functions were created. For example, PHARMAC, intended as the nation's drug purchaser

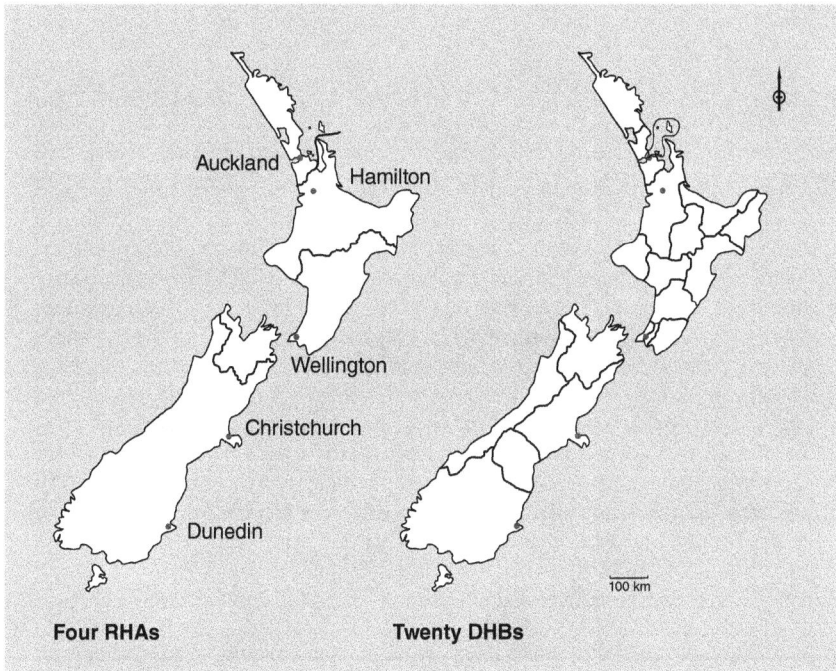

Figure 1.3 RHA and DHB maps.

and therefore a major influence on new medicines, was a creation of the four RHAs. A Public Health Commission saw a few years of life during this period while a National Health Committee advised the Minister. A vignette taken from Kathryn's field notes gives a sense of the frustrations of some people with haemophilia with this fragmented and marketised model of service.

Dividing care: haemophilia and the RHA system

At the beginning of our research in 1994, we spent some time piloting our research materials—questionnaires, focus groups, and interviews. As part of this process, Kathryn travelled to some provincial areas where people did not have immediate recourse to specialists and where outreach support was limited. In the process, she met with a middle-aged man with moderate haemophilia, whom we call Graeme, who had contracted hepatitis C through his treatment (see Box 1.1).

Under the RHA system, Graeme, a depressed man with haemophilia, hepatitis C, and chronic pain, is effectively lost in the maze that should lead to care. Because of his hepatitis C and haemophilia, he was obliged to attend the hospital for dental treatment as no dentist in his town was equipped to care for him. His haemophilia treatment was not coordinated with the rest

Box 1.1

Graeme's story

As a result of hepatitis C and (unsuccessful) treatment with interferon, Graeme described that he had become depressed and very tired. He had also experienced a bad reaction during treatment for an internal bleed a few years before. As a result, he was trying to avoid clotting factor replacement therapy. Graeme did not want to undertake home treatment, partly because of this reaction. He owned to being scared by it. He was on Accident Compensation Commission (ACC)[2] income support for an injury the treatment of which was complicated by haemophilia. This injury caused him pain as did a joint into which he had repeated bleeds, a 'target joint', which had become arthritic. Graeme was married, his wife worked nearby, and they lived in an area quite close to a small hospital in his local RHA area at which there was no haematologist. The nearest haematologist was at a larger CHE (hospital), a three-hour drive away, in a different Health Authority area so it was funded and administered separately. One bright spot in his story was the visit of the NZHS outreach worker a couple of weeks before Kathryn met Graeme. An edited version of Kathryn's notes and conversation is below.

> The hospital in another RHA with a haematologist send Graeme an appointment card about once a year. He thinks his local hospital would not be impressed [i.e., would be angry] if they knew. At his appointments, the haematologist checks his condition, his joints, does blood tests, but cannot send the results to Graeme's local hospital because there is no one there to send them to and Graeme believes that no one there is interested anyway.
>
> For dental work: Graeme said, 'I've got to go to the [local] hospital, infectious diseases department [because of Hepatitis C] to get [my teeth] done. But the hospital still charges me for it. I was wondering if ACC should be paying or if someone else should be paying? There is nowhere in town to get that sort of thing done.' When Kathryn asked if he had approached ACC, he replied, 'Well you have got to get that [authorisation] back from a doctor again, and nobody wants to sign a form for it'. He had not yet discussed it fully with his GP.

Kathryn asked if he would get a haemophilia treatment before his teeth were done. He replied, 'At the moment they would charge me probably for the treatment [laughs]. They send you a bill first, if you don't pay that you don't get an appointment.' It turned out that he had to pay to see the haematologist in the other RHA area as well, and also he had to pay for his own travel. He explained that ACC will not pay that because it is out of the area, and they only pay so many kilometres. Reportedly, the haematologist from the other RHA was willing to come up to do a clinic at the local hospital, but he was not allowed to because he worked in a different RHA area.

KATHRYN: But you don't have other options but to go out of the area!
GRAEME: No.

of his care. This is not simply a function of his living in a smallish regional city, although that is part of it. Rather it is because the RHA system inhibited good communication and shared care between the small centres and the larger ones where the necessary specialists worked. Everything that crossed an RHA boundary had to be paid for either by the patient or the other CHE. We were told by a doctor that even a phone call from a health professional asking for advice from another doctor in a different RHA had to be billed and there was a reluctance to reach out for advice because of this penalty. As a result, it was the patient who paid, literally and figuratively. Yet at this time, there were only four RHAs. The more fragmented health systems that preceded or ultimately followed the RHA system were even worse for people with haemophilia as even more boundaries were created. But even with only four bounded areas, some unfortunates like Graeme had to cross boundaries. Their experience of haemophilia was partially created by the divisions in the organisation of health care.

However, within the RHA system a quasi-national system for haemophilia was in the process of developing. One North Island RHA had been given the role by the other three RHA haematology services to coordinate aspects of haemophilia services and little by little a more national (rational) approach was in train. It did not have the ability to develop fully because of the abrupt restructuring that took place from 1997, but the seeds were sewn.

A national health system, and more fragmentation

Like the Area Health Board system that preceded it, the RHA structures hardly had time to shake down when once again a wholesale reorganisation took place. For a brief period (1997–2000) New Zealand had a single national health purchaser, the Health Funding Authority. The haemophilia community breathed a collective sigh of relief. The former CHEs returned once again to being Health and Hospital Services (HHS), no longer were compelled to make a profit, and were directed by appointed and elected Boards. But this relief was short-lived.

The final set of formal restructuring (to date) abolished this system in 2000, and created 21 District Health Boards (DHBs), which were once again both providers and purchasers (see Figure 1.3). These Boards also have elected and appointed members and are funded on a population base that covers primary and hospital care, mental health, and some disability services. The number of DHBs, subsequently decreased to 20, include three in Auckland, and two in Wellington, and many of the 'back room' functions have been amalgamated. Much of the policy setting was once again recentralised in the Ministry of Health.

The establishing act (Public Health and Disability Act 2000) allowed for primary health organisations that were designed partly on the not-for-profit trusts that emerged under the RHA system and also on some of the successful Independent Practitioners Associations. These PHOs or Primary

Health Organisations are not-for-profit, but are fund-holders for the various groups of community providers, e.g., GP clinics, Māori health care providers, and multidisciplinary primary care clinics that affiliate to them. Patients of these health care providers opt to enrol with a PHO specified by their provider. Initially, access funding was provided to heavily subsidise certain high need groups and children under six (Barnett and Barnett 2008; Gauld 2009). By 2014, most children under six visited their GPs at no cost during normal working hours and this provision was extended to age 13 mid-2015. Levels of subsidy, and the amounts patients paid differed based on the patient category and the practice. For example, at that time, an adult visiting a regular GP practice would pay on average $38, whereas one visiting a very low cost access GP practice would pay $15. In April 2014, the Ministry of Health reported that 94.9 per cent of the New Zealand population was enrolled in a PHO, and that there were 32 PHOs (Ministry of Health 2014).

During our final update study in 2005 and 2006, we encountered a number of individual arrangements devised to overcome the problem posed by the rare and expensive disorder of haemophilia to a fragmented health service with a limited number of specialists. Where patients in some DHB areas did not have access to specialist care, a shared care arrangement between two DHBs had been negotiated. In other cases, families got all their haemophilia care from another DHB because of various problems with their own DHB, and in complex situations, patients tended to end up in Christchurch, Wellington, or Auckland hospitals for care. All this of course meant that funds had to be remitted from one DHB to another. Two people we met had actually moved their place of residence to be in a DHB area where they perceived there was better care—a trend we had noted in earlier phases of the study. These individual decisions have serious implications for the population-funded DHB budgets. A family with haemophilia moving into the area unexpectedly, we were told, could bankrupt a small DHB. A popular joke was that it was cheaper for a DHB to buy a house for a haemophilic family in another DHB area than to treat them. At least we interpreted it as a joke. One positive change noted in this phase was the creation of a single New Zealand blood service to manage clotting factor produced from human blood and the single agency PHARMAC, which purchased the recombinant clotting factor products. These were and are important organisations for haemophilia care.

When our study began, the seven regional blood services were relatively separate. Our initial study showed that the combination of RHA funding models and regional blood service supply boundaries meant that there was inequitable access to haemophilia care and treatment across New Zealand, despite the best efforts of haematologists to overcome these divisions by sharing resources and cooperating wherever possible. This was not simply a rural-urban division. Some cities had sufficient product to treat preventatively while others did not. As a result, some boys grew up with undamaged joints and others did not; people in some areas were able to have elective surgery, others could not. Multiple problems of safety, supply, inefficiency, competition, poor communication, among other things, led to a review in 1996 and eventually to the formation of The New Zealand Blood Service, which is a statutory corporation with the Ministers of Finance and Health as shareholders (Park, Scott, and Benseman 1999).[3]

PHARMAC was established in June 1993 as a company owned by the RHAs that would centrally purchase and manage pharmaceuticals for community use. In 2001, it became a Crown entity. On its website, it lists as one of its milestones for 2005 'Centralised purchasing of haemophilia products produces savings of $30 million' (PHARMAC 2008). PHARMAC now has a crucial role to play in the haemophilia community.

Restructuring has not finished. Minor and major tweaks to the provision and funding of health and disability services are ongoing. In May 2018, the Minister of Health in the Labour coalition government announced a comprehensive review of the public health system. Alongside internal pressures for change in haemophilia management, external forces, such as negotiations of the Trans Pacific Partnership, which had the potential to increase the costs of treatment products purchased by PHARMAC, caused anxiety.

Also important to some members of the community are the social provisions for income maintenance, disability supplements for children, policies to reduce the incidental medical costs of chronic conditions (such as travel to hospital), domestic purposes benefits, superannuation, state housing affordability, and the like. Needless to say in the New Zealand context, several of these have been in a state of flux. The Accident Compensation Commission and its policies were also substantially restructured during this period with notable effect on people with haemophilia and especially those with hepatitis C (see chapters 5 and 6).

While these policy transformations were underway, the haemophilia community was also experiencing challenges and changes that had their origins elsewhere. Most notable and negative were the blood-borne viruses. As described earlier in this chapter, changes in treatment products, especially away from blood-derived products to genetically engineered synthetic clotting factor replacements, and the increasing availability of prophylactic treatment transformed the lives of people with haemophilia and their caregivers. Improvements in multidisciplinary care for haemophilia and in the treatment of the blood-borne viruses, the continual advocacy of HFNZ and its precursor, NZHS, with its Medical Advisors, to secure the best possible treatment and welfare for its members through its own efforts and working in partnership with others, also positively affected people's lives. These activities led to the instigation in 2006 of the National Haemophilia Management Group, which managed a single fund for a coordinated haemophilia service delivered by the DHBs. The story therefore is one of multiple and often intersecting changes. The origins of these changes range from global to local but they are embodied in the experience of people with haemophilia living in particular places and times in New Zealand. One of the strengths of an ethnographic study over time is that big issues, such as national health reforms, take on a graspable character when seen through the experiences of a particular community of interest. But it is well to remember that this is just one community of interest and a focus on other communities would produce other stories.

Organisation of the book

In chapter 2, we explore the narratives of the everyday experiences of people with haemophilia, attempting to bring to life different haemophilias as experienced over time. The chapter is organised in terms of the life course, with variations. One of the themes apparent in the narratives of people living with haemophilia, which pervades the other chapters, is the need for advocacy, and the building and embodiment of resilience and expertise. This is apparent at the microlevel of clinical encounters, in the wider community, and as an aspect of citizenship.

Ghannam and Sholkamy (2004, 1) argue that 'the strategies that men and women adopt to attain health and well-being are also expressions of identity'. They present experiences of health and illness in their studies in Egypt as 'sites of self and social expression that are charted on the landscape of the body'. Others, especially Crandon-Malamud (1993), also working in pluralistic health settings, have made the case for health-seeking strategies not being merely an expression of identity but part of how claims to identity are made. Using these ideas, in chapter 3, we focus particularly on haemophilia as both a sexed and gendered condition that is shaped by and contributes to the enactment of gendered identities and values in New Zealand. We show how key symbols of masculine and feminine identity in the New Zealand context, namely rugby and carrying/caring, are alive in the haemophilia context and how they are changing in tandem with broader societal changes. We argue that the enactment of sex/gender in this context is part of the creation of local biologies of haemophilia.

This theme is taken up again in chapter 4 where new technologies in the treatment of haemophilia have led to new haemophilias. We are working with a concept of technologies as assemblages that consist of networked material objects, systems of knowledge, conventional practices, and the meanings with which they are imbued, together creating apparently coherent entities. In this usage of technologies, we follow the work of Latour (1987), Brodwin (2000), and others, who focus on how materiality and meaning are interconnected at key points in science and technology. After a consideration of changing treatment technologies and their implications, we examine genetic testing, especially carrier testing, prenatal testing and preimplantation technologies, and how these have created new demands for moral reasoning for parents and potential parents, and new dilemmas for differently situated members of the haemophilia community. According to Brodwin (2000), and as we discovered in our research, the value and meaning of technologies are created through their social life, which may encompass people and groups who never participate in these technologies but for whom they are meaningful nonetheless.

Social suffering (Kleinman, Das, and Lock 1997) of individuals and the community of people with haemophilia in relation to hepatitis C, and their responses in terms of advocacy for rights, recognition and equity are the foci of chapters 5 and 6. In chapter 5, we chart the stories of the blood-borne viruses, hepatitis B, HIV and AIDS, and hepatitis C, focussing most particularly on the individual and community experiences. In partial contrast, chapter 6 is a study of HFNZ and draws on the literature of governmentality (Rose 1999; Rose and Novas 2005), partnership, and public participation (Young 2000). The transformation of a small support group into HFNZ provides the background to our examination of two case studies. One concerns the blood-borne viruses and the achievement of a negotiated settlement with the Crown of the long-outstanding hepatitis C affair in 2008. The other is the changing relationships between HFNZ, haemophilia medical specialists, the Ministry of Health and the local health authorities, and particularly the advocacy process that led to a national haemophilia service in 2006–7. This also entailed the changing relationships between the Foundation, the Blood Service, multinational pharmaceutical companies, and PHARMAC. Chapter 6 provides a case study of the intricacies of the intersection of social citizenship and active citizenship (Humpage 2015).

Our concluding chapter, chapter 7, first draws on the personal experiences of two authors, Mike and Deon, to overview different haemophilias before, during, and after our active research period and looks forward to the future. Finally, Kathryn and Julie reflect on the research and its contribution to understanding local biologies of haemophilia, to medical anthropology, and to providing insights into local and international social issues.

Notes

1. Single quote marks with no source indicate that the phrase is commonly used by people in the haemophilia community and can be found in many ethnographic fieldnotes and transcripts, as in 'You just deal with it!', a statement of stoic coping.
2. ACC is fully explained in chapter 5. It was set up in the 1970s to compensate all people in New Zealand for accidental injury, in exchange for citizens foregoing the right to sue. It is funded by levies on employers and employees, but covers everybody, including tourists. ACC covers some or all health costs, and may also compensate for loss of income.
3. It started life as a CHE in 1998 and then an HHS (http://www.nzblood.co.nz/?t=34).

References

Agar, M. 1980. *The Professional Stranger: An Informal Introduction to Anthropology*. New York: Academic Press.

Anderson, B. 1991 [1983]. *Imagined Communities: Reflections on the Origin and Spread of Nationalism*. London: Verso.

Ashton, T. 2005. 'Recent Developments in the Funding and Organisation of the New Zealand Health System'. *Australia and New Zealand Health Policy* 2:9. doi:10.1186/1743-8462-2-9.

Ballara, A. 1998. *Iwi: The Dynamics of Māori Tribal Organisation from c.1769 to c.1945*. Wellington: Victoria University Press.

Barnett, R., and P. Barnett. 2008. 'Reinventing Primary Care: The New Zealand Case Compared'. In *Primary Health Care: People, Practice, Place*, edited by V. Crooks and G. Andrews, 149–65. London: Ashgate.

Belich, J. 2001. *Paradise Reforged. A History of the New Zealanders from the 1880s to the Year 2000*. Honolulu: University of Hawai'i Press.

Belich, J., and L. Wevers. 2008. 'Understanding New Zealand Cultural Identities'. Discussion Paper prepared by the Stout Research Centre for New Zealand Studies for the Ministry of Culture and Heritage. Wellington: Victoria University.

Bell, R., M. Kawharu, K. Taylor, M. Belgrave, and P. Meihana. 2017. *The Treaty on the Ground: Where We Are Headed and Why It Matters*. Auckland: Massey University Press.

Blank, R.H. 1994. *New Zealand Health Policy: A Comparative Study*. Auckland: Oxford University Press.

Bourdieu, P. *et al.* 1999. *The Weight of the World: Social Suffering in Contemporary Society*. Translated by P.P. Ferguson, S. Emanuel, J. Johnson, and S.T. Waryn. Cambridge: Polity Press.

Brodwin, P. 2000. 'Introduction'. In *Biotechnology and Culture: Bodies, Anxieties, Ethics*, edited by P. Brodwin, 1–26. Bloomington: Indiana University Press.

Brown, S.A., J. Phillips, C. Barnes, J. Curtin, S. McRae, P. Ockelford, J. Rowell, M.P. Smith, and S. Dunkley. 2015. 'Challenges in Hemophilia Care in Australia and New Zealand'. *Current Medical Research and Opinion* 31 (11). doi:10.1185%2F030007995.2015.108

Carnahan, M.J. 2013. *Allies or Enemies: How Those Needing Help Learned to Help Themselves in the Face of Bad Blood*. Christchurch: Haemophilia Foundation of New Zealand.

Cheung, J. 2007. *Wealth Disparities in New Zealand*. Wellington: Statistics New Zealand.

Clement, P. 2014. 'Joint Diseases, Prophy and Microbleeds: Are We Doing Enough?' *PEN* 21(2):1 &7–12.

Cohen, A. 1985. *The Symbolic Construction of Community*. London: Routledge.

Crandon-Malamud, L. 1993. *From the Fat of Our Souls: Social Change, Political Process, and Medical Pluralism in Bolivia*. Berkeley: University of California Press.

di Leonardo, M. 1991. 'Introduction. Gender, Culture and Political Economy: Feminist Anthropology in Historical Perspective'. In *Gender at the Crossroads of Knowledge: Feminist Anthropology in the Postmodern Era*, edited by M. di Leonardo, 1–48. Berkeley: California University Press.

Dyck, N. 2000. 'Home Field Advantage?' In *Constructing the Field: Ethnographic Fieldwork in the Contemporary World*, edited by V. Amit, 32–53. London and New York: Routledge.

Farmer, P. 1992. *AIDS and Accusation: Haiti and the Geography of Blame*. Berkeley: University of California Press.

Fassin, D. 2007. *When Bodies Remember: Experiences and Politics of AIDS in South Africa*. Berkeley: University of California Press.

Fischer, D.H. 2012. *Fairness and Freedom: A History of Two Open Societies, New Zealand and the United States*. Oxford: Oxford University Press.

Fitzgerald, R. 2004. 'The New Zealand Health Reforms: Dividing the Labour of Care'. *Social Science and Medicine* 58 (2):331–41.

Gauld, R. 2009. *The New Health Policy*. Maidenhead: Open University Press.

Ghannam, H., and F. Sholkamy, eds. 2004. *Health and Identity in Egypt: Shifting Frontiers*. Cairo: American University in Cairo.

Gibbs, A., D. Fraser, and J. Scott. 1988. 'Unshackling the Hospitals: Report of the Hospitals and Related Services Taskforce'. Wellington: Government Print.

[HFNZ] Haemophilia Foundation of New Zealand. 2016a. 'Bleeding Disorders–Haemophilia'. http://www.haemophilia.org.nz/bleeding-disorders/haemophilia (last accessed 11 Nov, 2018).

———. 2016b. 'Inhibitors'. http://www.haemophilia.org.nz/bleeding-disorders/complications-associated-with-haemophilia/#Inhibitors (last accessed 11 Nov, 2018).

Hammersley, A., and P. Atkinson. 1983. *Ethnography: Principles in Practice*. London: Tavistock Publications.

Haworth, N. 1994. 'Neoliberalism, Economic Internationalisation and the Contemporary State in New Zealand'. In *Leap into the Dark: The Changing Role of the State in New Zealand since 1984*, edited by A. Sharp, 19–40. Auckland: Auckland University Press.

Howden-Chapman, P., S. Bierre, and C. Cunningham. 2013. 'Building Inequality'. In *Inequality: A New Zealand Crisis*, edited by M. Rashbrooke, 105–19. Wellington: Bridget Williams Books.

Howden-Chapman, P., J. Park, K. Scott, and J. Carter. 1996. 'An Intimate Reliance: Health Reform, Viral Infections and the Safety of Blood Products'. In *Intimate Details and Vital Statistics*, edited by P. Davis, 168–84. Auckland: Auckland University Press.

Humpage, L. 2015. *Policy Change, Public Attitudes and Social Citizenship: Does Neoliberalism Matter?* Bristol: Policy Press.

Joint Regional Health Authority Project Team. 1996. 'Joint Regional Health Authority Project: Purchasing and Provision of Haemophilia Services'. Final Report. [no publication data].

Jutel, A.G. 2011. *Putting a Name to It: Diagnosis in Contemporary Society*. Baltimore: Johns Hopkins University Press.

Kawharu, M. 2013. 'Whakapapa and Metamorphosis'. *SITES (NS)* 10 (1):51–72.

Kelsey, J. 1997. *The New Zealand Experiment: A World Model for Structural Adjustment?* Auckland: Auckland University Press/Bridget Williams Books.

Kirp, D. 1999. 'Look Back in Anger: Hemophilia and AIDS Activism in the International Tainted-Blood Crisis'. *Journal of Comparative Policy Analysis: Research and Practice* 1:177–202.

Kleinman, A., V. Das, and M. Lock. 1997. 'Introduction'. In *Social Suffering*, edited by Kleinman, A., V. Das, and M. Lock, ix–xxvii. Berkeley: University of California Press.

Latour, B. 1987. *Science in Action: How to Follow Scientists and Engineers Through Society*. Cambridge: Harvard University Press.

Laugesen, M., and R. Gauld. 2012. *Democratic Governance in Health*. Dunedin: Otago University Press.

Lock, M. 2001. 'The Tempering of Medical Anthropology: Troubling Natural Categories'. *Medical Anthropology Quarterly* 15 (4):478–92.

Lynch, B. 2015. 'New Zealand and Asia-Pacific Integration: Sailing the Waka in Ever-widening Circles'. Discussion Paper 17/15 for the Centre for Strategic Studies, Wellington: Victoria University of Wellington.

McClure, M. 1998. *A Civilised Community: A History of Social Security in New Zealand 1898–1998*. Auckland: Auckland University Press/Historical Branch, Department of Internal Affairs.

McKenzie, A. 1997. 'Workfare: The New Zealand Experience and Future Directions'. *Social Policy Journal of New Zealand Te Puna Whakaaro* 8. https://www.msd.govt.nz/about-msd-and-our-work/publications-resources/journals-and-magazines/social-policy-journal/spj08/workfare-new-zealand-experience-and-future-directions.html

Ministry of Health. 2014. 'About Primary Health Organisations'. www.health.govt.nz (last accessed 11 Nov, 2018).

Mol, A. 2002. *The Body Multiple: Ontology in Medical Practice*. Durham: Duke University Press.

Nairn, K., J. Higgins, and J. Sligo. 2012. *Children of Rogernomics: A Neoliberal Generation Leaves School*. Dunedin: Otago University Press.

Ockelford, P., A.G. Benny, N.S. Van de Water, and E. Berry. 1989. 'Haemophilia Management in New Zealand'. *New Zealand Medical Journal* 102:189–91.

OECD. 2014. *Focus on Inequality and Growth-December 2014*. www.oecd.org/social/inequality-and-poverty.htm (last accessed 11 Nov, 2018).

Okma, K.G.H., and L. Crivelli. 2010. 'Six Countries, Six Reform Models: The Healthcare Reform Experience of Israel, The Netherlands, New Zealand, Singapore, Switzerland and Taiwan: Healthcare Reforms "Under the Radar Screen" '. *JAMA* 304 (18)2067–71.

Park, J. 1992. Research Partnerships: A Discussion Paper Based on Case Studies from 'The Place of Alcohol in the Lives of New Zealand Women' Project. *Women's Studies International Forum* 15 (5&6):581–91.

Park, J., K. Scott, J. Benseman, and E. Berry. 1995. *A Bleeding Nuisance: Living with Haemophilia in Aotearoa New Zealand*. Auckland: Department of Anthropology, University of Auckland.

Park, J., K. Scott, and J. Benseman. 1999. 'Dealing with a Bleeding Nuisance: A Study of Haemophilia Care in New Zealand'. *New Zealand Medical Journal* 112:155–58.

Park, J., and B. Strookappe. 1996. 'Deciding about Having Children in Families with Haemophilia'. *New Zealand Journal of Disability Studies* 3:51–67.

Park, J., and D. York. 2008. *The Social Ecology of New Technologies and Haemophilia in New Zealand: 'A Bleeding Nuisance' Revisited*. RAL 8. Auckland: Department of Anthropology, University of Auckland. https://researchspace.auckland.ac.nz/handle/2292/4534 (last accessed Nov 11, 2018).

Peyvandi, F., and I. Garagiola. 2015. 'Treatment of Hemophilia in the Near Future'. *Seminars in Thrombosis and Hemostasis* 4 (8):838–48.

PHARMAC. 2008. 'History'. www.pharmac.govt.nz/dhbs/AboutPHARMAC/history (last accessed 11 Nov, 2018).

———. 2015. 'Haemophilia Treatments'. https://www.pharmac.govt.nz/medicines/my-medicine-has-changed/haemophilia-treatments/ (last accessed 11 Nov, 2018).

Prince, R., R. Kearns, and D. Craig. 2006. 'Governmentality, Discourse and Space in the New Zealand Health Care System, 1991–2003'. *Health & Place* 12 (3):253–66.

Pruthi, R.K. 2005. 'Hemophilia: A Practical Approach to Genetic Testing'. *Mayo Clinic Proceedings* 80 (11):1485–99.

Rabinow, P. 1996. *Essays on the Anthropology of Reason*. Princeton, NJ: Princeton University Press.

Rashbrooke, M. 2013. 'Inequality and New Zealand'. In *Inequality: A New Zealand Crisis*, edited by M. Rashbrooke, 20–36. Wellington: Bridget Williams Books.

Reid, P. 2015. 'Promoting Health Equity'. In *Promoting Health in Aotearoa New Zealand*, edited by L. Signal and M. Ratima, 146–161. Dunedin: Otago University Press.

Resnik, S. 1999. *Blood Saga: Hemophilia, AIDS, and the Survival of a Community*. Berkeley: University of California Press.

Roberts, H. R., and M. R. Jones. 1990. 'Disorders of Hemostasis: Congenital Disorders of Blood Coagulations Factors. Hemophilia and Related Conditions'. In *Hematology*, 4th ed, edited by W. Williams, E. Beutler, A. Erslev, and M. Lichtman, 1453–1753. New York: McGraw-Hill.

Rose, N. 1999. *Powers of Freedom: Reframing Political Thought*. Cambridge: Cambridge University Press.

Rose, N., and C. Novas. 2005. 'Biological Citizenship'. In *Global Assemblages: Technology, Politics, and Ethics as Anthropological Problems*, edited by A. Ong and S. J. Collier, 439–63. Oxford: Blackwell Publishing.

Rosendaal, F.R., C. Smit, and E. Briet. 1991. 'Hemophilia Treatment in Historical Perspective: A Review of Medical and Social Developments'. *Annals of Hematology* 62:5–15.

Royal Commission on Social Policy. 1988. *The April Report. The Royal Commission on Social Policy*. Wellington: The Royal Commission.

Scott, K. 1997. 'Haemophilia Care Not Just the Domain of Specialists'. *New Zealand Family Physician* 24 (5):16–8.

———. 2013. 'The Politics of Influence: An Anthropological Analysis of Collective Political Action in Contemporary Democracy'. PhD diss. in Anthropology. Auckland: University of Auckland.

Signal, L., and M. Ratima. 2015. *Promoting Health in Aotearoa New Zealand*. Dunedin: Otago University Press.

Statistics New Zealand. 2015. 'New Zealand in Profile: 2014'. www.stats.govt.nz/browse_for_stats/snapshots-of-nz/nz-in-profile-2014.aspx (last accessed 11 Nov, 2018).

Strathern, M. 1987. 'The Limits of Auto-anthropology'. In *Anthropology at Home*, edited by A. Jackson, 59–67. London: Tavistock.

Strookappe, B. 1996. 'My Fifty-Fifty Chance: The Social Implications of Carrying the Haemophilia Gene'. Master of Arts Thesis in Anthropology. University of Auckland.

Taylor, G., and M.P. Power. 2011. *Risk, Science and Blood: Politics, HIV, Hepatitis and Haemophilia in Ireland*. Galway: ARAN, Access to Research at NUI Galway. http://hdl.handle.net/10379/2547 (last accessed 11 Nov, 2018).

Trnka, S., and L. McLauchlan. 2012. 'Becoming "Half A Doctor": Parent-Experts and the Normalisation of Childhood Asthma in Aotearoa/New Zealand'. *SITES (NS)* 9 (2):3–22.

Woodward, A., and T. Blakely. 2014. *The Healthy Country: A History of Life & Death in New Zealand*. Auckland: Auckland University Press.

World Federation of Hemophilia. 2012. 'Carriers and Women with Hemophilia'. https://www.wfh.org/en/abd/carriers/carriers-and-women-with-hemophilia-en (last accessed 11 Nov, 2018).

———. 2015. 'History of the WFH'. https://www.wfh.org/en/about-us/50-years-of-advancing-treatment-for-all (last accessed 11 Nov, 2018).

Young, I.M. 2000. *Inclusion and Democracy*. Oxford: Oxford University Press.

2 'Pretty normal really'

Different haemophilias: an introduction

What's it like having haemophilia? We researchers would seldom directly ask this of a person, yet here we attempt to provide some answers. 'Answers' has to be plural because, despite the commonalities of having an inherited condition, either haemophilia A or B, there are as many different haemophilias as there are people with it.[1] The answers go beyond haemophilia as a medical condition to include holistic aspects of being.

In this chapter, we want to convey what makes up haemophilia for each individual and each family: what are the outcomes of the interactions of the specific genes with what we might broadly call the exigencies of life? Despite haemophilia A and B being single-gene disorders,[2] we want to move away from the presumption that haemophilia is the same condition globally with just minor variations. In anthropology as in genetic sciences, epigenetic phenomena increasingly have been recognised as having lifelong modulating interactions with genes. Whether epigenetics is defined narrowly in terms of the 'heritable chemical modifications to DNA' (Thayer and Non 2015, 722), the role of noncoding DNA in the expression and modulation of genes, or broadly in terms of developmental systems theory (Lock and Nguyen 2010, 335), it has forged new thinking about the human genome. Genetics and epigenetics together interacting over time in open systems with the exigencies of life in a particular time and place create the condition experienced as haemophilia.

People with haemophilia and those caring for them explained to us that although there were internationally recognised levels of severity, these did not correlate precisely with the intensity or number of bleeds. Individuals with the same severity level also experienced different degrees of arthropathy, skeletal, muscle, and nerve damage. Even in a single individual, blood chemistry appeared to change, making bleeds more likely at some times than at others. Men and women with low factor levels also had different experiences. For example, some women experienced very severe menstrual bleeding, and recent evidence suggests that women carriers of mutations for haemophilia show evidence of joint damage from an early age (CDC 2015). To complicate matters further, some people with haemophilia also have another condition that disrupts clotting: von Willebrand disease. Unlike haemophilia, this genetic disorder is inherited equally by men and women. People with von Willebrand disease are now included in Haemophilia Foundation of New Zealand (HFNZ) but unless they also have haemophilia they are not included in our research.

The experiences of haemophilia in New Zealand, a moderately well-off country with a public health system, are different from those in other countries. In a country like the United States, that is wealthier and spends more on health care but has a sparse public health system despite federally funded haemophilia centres, about 30 per cent of the population may miss out on adequate treatment. Rapidly developing countries with great inequality, such as India, may reach less than 20 per cent of the haemophilia population (Hemophilia Federation India 2014; Phadke 2011). Within New Zealand, as this chapter details, individuals' haemophilias are dependent on the type of mutation, certainly, but also on social and technological changes over generations, the organisation of health and associated cares, stigmatising or inclusive practices of groups and organisations, and characteristics such as gender, class, and ethnicity. In the twenty-first century in well-served countries, haemophilia is often seen as a not very serious problem. Children with it usually experience little educational disruption as part of their haemophilia. No longer does the fear of HIV and AIDS hover over every infusion of replacement clotting factor. Pain is not a constant inevitable consequence of having haemophilia. Yet learning that one has haemophilia even in the twenty-first century may be emotionally fraught. We approach haemophilia as a multidimensional cultural phenomenon with implications for most aspects of life from infancy to old age.

Given this multiplicity, a chapter devoted to the local biology of haemophilia in New Zealand over several generations presents some challenges. In response we have organised our narratives according to a generalised life course framework, integrating diverse dimensions along the way. We begin with an analysis of narratives of finding out about haemophilia through an initial diagnosis, which usually occurs early in life, then proceed through life stages. The narratives from the three different study periods are woven together, but are identified in terms of their dates of reference. Our studies themselves have spanned two decades, but the narrative time depth is greater, as our participants retold events up to 50 years before 1995. Our account is based primarily on interviews with people with haemophilia and the parents of children with it, because, as much as possible, we want to convey the sense of people's own stories and phrases. It is supported by our understandings gained from our varied involvements in the haemophilia community, from our readings of the literature, and, for two of us, by being men with haemophilia born a generation apart.

The life story approach used in our interviews and our attention to the social context of Aotearoa New Zealand enabled us to identify different haemophilias and to scrutinise New Zealand society and culture through a haemophilia lens. Through our long-term engagement we can show, for example, that as a result of changing social norms about inclusivity and more effective treatment, parents are no longer as worried about their children's schooling. But concerns about serious injury, keeping veins 'good', participation in sports—especially rugby—and being a parent-expert-caregiver remain. We see, too, that recognition within the haemophilia community of the diverse needs and identities of members is part of a broader social movement, and that approaches to adversity, such as a determination to 'cope', have much in common through the generations.

Research narratives

Narratives are ways of making sense of and giving meaning to experience, as Garro and Mattingly (2000), Kleinman (1988), and others have discussed. They may be very brief or take hours in the telling. Often at the end of a narrative, or mininarrative within a longer story, there may be a phrase summing up one of the key themes, e.g.: 'He wouldn't be the great guy he is without haemophilia'. Such reflections often convey a moral evaluation. After detailing her son's struggles with haemophilia, this mother explained that she would not wish haemophilia on anyone but was proud of how her son had dealt with it, and proud of him. Narratives also demonstrate a person's sense of perspective and identity, and in haemophilia narratives, there is often a tendency to espouse stoicism and to downplay the condition. Narratives foresee futures and can convey hope. The narrative of continually improving, safe treatment options explains why a father in 2005 is not too worried about having a carrier daughter: 'Maybe when my daughter grows up and has children, you'll just need to take a pill once a month for haemophilia'.

Diagnosis is often a key point in a narrative. It can be a relief: the end of something, namely a general or specific worry, and the beginning of something new, namely learning about living with haemophilia. How a diagnosis is received depends on the narrative in which the parent or patient is enmeshed. For families with a known history of haemophilia, diagnosis may come as the confirmation of what they had suspected and were already familiar with. But it still may mean that hopes of beating the odds are dashed. In families where there was no family history of haemophilia, observations of their child's excessive bruising often provoked anxiety about the child having leukaemia. In this often secret narrative of possible leukaemia, diagnosis was not just the relief of knowing, but the relief of thinking it was not as serious as leukaemia, as this mother said in 1995: 'Before the diagnosis, I thought it was leukaemia and I was so relieved to learn it was only haemophilia'. But in the context of parental narratives about a perfect newborn, diagnosis can be devastating (Buchbinder and Timmermans 2011). Another mother in 1995 said: 'I just remember crying for about two weeks solid, just this whole thing about what was going to happen to my baby, what does the future hold?'. For other parents, receiving a diagnosis of haemophilia meant that the suspicion that they were abusing their child was lifted and they could see a way forward. In her detailed study of diagnosis, Jutel (2011, 1) suggested that 'Receiving a diagnosis is like being handed a road map in the middle of a forest. It shows the way but not necessarily the way out'. For many in the haemophilia community, diagnosis was the way out, but how hard that road would be was not clearly depicted. Additionally, not all diagnoses were straightforward.

Diagnosis is both the process and the outcome of establishing what the matter is, and, where possible, what is causing the problem. Its purpose is to provide a basis for what to do and some sense of what the future might hold: a plan for action and a prognosis. All these elements of a diagnosis have varied meanings and are embedded in different narratives for the people involved: the newly diagnosed and their parents, grandparents and other family members, haematologists, paediatricians, geneticists, haemophilia nurses, physiotherapists, and members of the other helping professions. But these disparate meanings are held together by the single definitive diagnosis: haemophilia A or B. A diagnosis for a condition that is well understood like haemophilia provides an explanation of cause, the narrative of genes, mutations, inheritance, and the clotting cascade, but it does not, and cannot, explain the existential question of 'Why me?'.

Where an illness begins is created through narrative, as in this story of a mother's curse that explained why there was haemophilia in one particular family: 'My grandfather emigrated from England. His mother didn't want him to [emigrate] and she cursed him. That's where the haemophilia started'. Meanings and values are created, reinforced, and promulgated through such narratives. They extend well beyond diagnosis and very often include moral messages. For example, stories about the decisions made by other people about specific issues, such as treatment options, or the choice of outdoor activities for boys with haemophilia, or testing of girls, and prenatal genetic testing very often included a summary statement of ethical values phrased along the lines of: 'If it is all right for the family, then it is all right'. This ethic of withholding judgement and tolerating plural values was part of the glue that held a diverse cross section of New Zealanders with different values, but shared haemophilia, together.

The relationship between narrative and experience is a contested domain in ordinary social life as well as in many academic and professional disciplines. How much does a story owe to the available narrative structures, the 'ready mades' (Bönisch-Brednich 2002), and how much is it an individual account of a person's experience of what happened? What is left out? What differences do retellings in different contexts make? How can we understand other people's stories? As Good and Good (1994, 140) explained, an understanding response to another's narrative is based to some extent on an imputation of shared experience: grief, joy, enjoying a laugh. But experience, like narrative, is culturally and situationally grounded. These uncertainties make narratives a lively area of debate within anthropology and related disciplines. Narrative analysis is necessarily open-ended.

Our approach in this research is based on the concept that people actively construct their worlds and themselves in the stories that they tell themselves and others. Therefore, analysis of narratives is a way to reach some understanding of those worlds and selves, as well as the events, experiences, and memories through which the narratives are expressed. Yet, because narratives are always elicited in and by a context, a reflexive awareness of this context needs to be part of the analysis. The narratives created through the 'living with haemophilia' research were coproduced by the research participants and the researchers and contain many complexities, such as participants' accounts of internal dialogues, renditions of dialogues with or between others, life stories and illness narratives, and interchanges with the interviewer. Typically, our conversations with participants about various topics would begin with an invitation such as, 'Tell me about…', or 'How have things been going since we last spoke?'. Some narratives on which we draw, such as those told at meetings and social gatherings, or written in books and newsletters, are independent of the researchers, and responsive to other contexts.

Narratives frame local biology, as in this example where a family and their medical specialists were trying to find a beginning for haemophilia in their family. The young mother, who herself had just been diagnosed as a carrier, and her son with haemophilia, said:

> 'Mother rang and said, "I am your time bomb".' She had just found out that she was a haemophilia carrier, which 'explained' how her daughter's son had haemophilia. This grandmother felt that the buck stopped with her.
>
> (Julie's notes after a recorded interview, 1995)

This narrative fragment suggests that the grandmother felt responsible for her grandson's haemophilia and her daughter's carrier status. It implied that haemophilia was a very serious condition that had exploded into her grandchild's generation. But there is more to the story. The grandmother's doctor had rung her with the test results and had said, 'You are the time bomb', creating a situation in which guilt or responsibility could flourish. The daughter was horrified at this implication, and tried to assure her mother that she was not responsible for their predicament.[3] With the potential emotional and intergenerational impact of diagnosis in mind, we now turn to more detailed case studies.

Learning haemophilia

As was often the case, Kathryn began the tape-recorded part of the research conversation in 1995 by asking Gillian[4] about her experience of 'finding out about haemophilia' and what had happened since. Gillian was the mother of a little girl who was six at the time of this research visit to their home. The girl had low clotting factor levels (see Box 2.1).

Box 2.1

Not to worry

I think she would have been only a couple of months old when she was treated for a haematoma (a big bruise). Yeah, she was still in a bassinet…, so I went to the GP, and he said that it was *'nothing to worry about'*. She obviously had banged something and that's how it happened. And I said, well, you know, I mean she's an infant. She can't move or roll over by herself or anything. I fail to see how she could hurt herself. But he said, 'Oh no, it's *nothing to worry about'*, and then, a couple of weeks after that she vomited up some blood and it was a very, very minute amount and I went to the after-hours surgery and they said there was *'nothing wrong with her*, she wasn't bleeding internally, and you know, *not to worry about it'*. And then when she was about 8 months old, she fell out of the walker onto a rock garden and hit her temple in the corner of her eye and she had a huge bruise and a big black eye and it was really quite nasty. And I went to the GP again and he said, 'No it's *nothing to worry* about'. It didn't need stitches or anything, it was fine. And so by the time she started presenting with all these bruises, we just thought, well you know, *because the GP wasn't worried, we weren't worried*.

And then when she was 13 months old, I had a new Plunket nurse and my GP was on holiday and there was a locum in. And the Plunket nurse looked at her and thought she had leukaemia and didn't say that to me though, just said: 'Had the doctor seen her?'. And I said, 'Yes, *he's not worried* about the bruises, he said that it's just ….'

And she said, 'Well I'd like him to have another look at this fresh batch of bruises.' So we went down…and the locum looked at her and thought that she was being abused. And questioned me about who was the care-giver and blah blah blah. And which I think was really good of that doctor that he was so diligent because otherwise it would have just gone on and on. And he sent her for a series of blood tests and they came back that she had haemophilia.

… He rang up and said he'd like to see us, to talk to us, and he was actually fantastic. I've never seen him since, he was just a locum. And he suggested that we get as much reading material from the library as we could on haemophilia before we saw the specialist and he'd made an appointment with the specialist at the public [hospital]. My husband was just really relieved that she didn't have leukaemia, cos he'd been thinking that's what it was, and I just didn't think anything. I mean the only thing I knew about haemophilia was the Russian Tsar had it and you know it was [inherited] in the family. I didn't know anything else and the following week we saw the head of pathology… and he explained the situation to us and basically they didn't know a lot, about the fact that she was a female. Didn't know what would happen. The worse scenario was when she reached puberty she'd have a hysterectomy and the best scenario was that nothing would happen, she'd be perfectly all right. But basically *'not to worry'* and if we needed any blood [treatment products] to come into hospital, to go to the children's ward. And we sort of left with the impression that if she had a car accident we'd have to be really careful, but apart from that—we sort of really had no idea.

Then the week after that she fell down the back steps onto some concrete and gave herself a terrible knock on the middle of her forehead. And we rushed her into hospital and very lucky that she was diagnosed when she was, because it could have been quite disastrous. And, yeah, we've been in and out of the hospital ever since really.

The modelling of 'not worrying' by the health professionals to Gillian, and her response is very striking: 'because the GP wasn't worried, we weren't worried'. She was not quite accurate in using 'we'. Gillian's husband, as well as the Plunket[5] nurse, had been quietly worried about leukaemia, because of the bruises, but they had not told Gillian, protecting her from worry. The professional respect relationship between the GP and the new Plunket nurse meant the nurse had not acted on her fears. But the locum's checking out his suspicion of child abuse provided the nurse with an opportunity to speak out and to encourage blood tests. The age and established practice of the GP, the toddler's gender, and the lack of experience of the parents at this time in the parent-patient role created a situation that would not necessarily be repeated as the parents grew into expert-parent-caregivers, as often happens when the condition is long-term (Trnka 2017, 56; Trnka and McLauchlan 2012).

The advice 'not to worry' pervades the story, except when the new nurse and locum doctor decide there is something to worry about: not child abuse after all, not leukaemia, but haemophilia. Suddenly, there is a flurry of activity. Once in the care of the specialist there is, again, nothing to worry about: there is treatment available, blood (products), directly from the children's ward, not via the often-tortuous route of Accident and Emergency. But really, there *is* something to worry about. Although haemophilia may be routinised, it can be 'quite disastrous' if accidents happen,[6] as they will, and the blood products themselves were a big worry because of recent viral contamination.

Telling the story five years after these events, Gillian used 'not to worry' phrases as structuring devices in her narrative, injecting some low-key humour. Arranged chronologically around repeated episodes of false reassurance, little stories exist within the larger narrative. They reach a dramatic climax where, had a health professional not worried and taken steps, the little girl would have later had a life threatening cerebral bleed when she fell head first onto concrete.

Gillian and Kathryn were complicit in the interview in knowing that there had been something to worry about all along, and that her family doctor had been overly intent on reassuring Gillian in this extremely unusual situation of a girl with severe haemophilia; a situation that even a specialist might miss. Gillian had known right from the beginning that there was something to worry about: a baby of a few months cannot injure herself in that way. But her parental experience-based knowledge had been brushed aside in an attempt to reassure. The right sort of care was provided by the locum who investigated child abuse and got tests done, and then set the family on the uneven path toward living with haemophilia.

Health system restructuring hardly figured in this narrative. As the first port of call, the GP has remained a constant presence, although considerable reorganising has happened with GP care too. The family lived in a city with a well-respected haemophilia service. The hospital-based specialist who eventually cared for this girl had his own pathway through secondary care for children with haemophilia: they avoided Accident and Emergency, the normal entry for acute problems, and went straight to the children's ward where there would not be delays in treatment through arguments about whether the child had haemophilia.

It is very unusual for girls to have such low factor levels because of haemophilia. Haematology texts at the time tended to write about haemophilia only in terms of boys, and therefore the difficulties described in arriving at the diagnosis might be considered exceptional. But it is not unusual for haemophilia diagnoses to take a long time in the 30 per cent of families where there has been no known previous history, as was the case in Gillian's family, and in the next narrative 10 years later, which is about a four-year-old boy, Uri, and his mother, Ursula (Park and York 2008, 7).

This 2005 narrative was set in a different part of New Zealand and under a restructured health system. By the time of the interview, it was the DHB system, but at diagnosis the National Health Authority had just replaced the RHA system. Julie and Ursula met at the town library for the interview as Ursula had come into town from a rural district for the day.

Four years before this interview, when Uri was eight months old, a very small accident had led to serious bleeding and eventually to a diagnosis of severe haemophilia. Before this his obvious bruises had been assessed as normal. The family lived near a city with a large hospital but were referred to their closest smaller hospital first. Ursula explained:

> … but he cut his finger and it bled and bled and bled, and then I took him to a doctor who said he must have cut an artery. I didn't think [so], it was just a little nick. So, the next time, he again had an injury and I took him to the GP and the GP said, 'This time we'd better test him', so they went and did a blood test and the person doing the blood test was quite incompetent and couldn't find a vein and poked around for quite some time and then got somebody else to do it, but in the meantime, had done quite a bit of damage. By the next morning, Uri had a bleed from his arm down to his fingers, a large bleed from all the [needle] holes. So that was our first one. He was immediately admitted to hospital because he was really unwell and unfortunately the paediatrician there didn't send him immediately to [City haemophilia centre],

where he should have been, and gave him a blood transfusion, which shouldn't have happened. And that was our first introduction, it was pretty horrific! But once we were hooked into the [haemophilia centre] carers, it's been brilliant ever since. They knew what they were doing. They had a really good haemophilia nurse at that time, and the care we received from then on was wonderful.

In this case it was the regular GP who picked up that there was something unusual about the baby's response, but only after initially discounting Ursula's observation that this was abnormal bleeding from a little nick. Although a paediatrician was involved, he was not a haematologist and perhaps did not initially consider a diagnosis of haemophilia. It was not until they were referred to the nearby haematology and oncology ward in a larger hospital that targeted treatment could begin. The staff there 'knew what they were doing'. In such situations, parents have to be strong advocates for their children. Later in Ursula's story she describes how she drove the 100 kilometres to the haemophilia centre after Uri had an accident on play equipment, rather than take him to a local hospital.

These two narratives about the long road to good care are replicated in various forms throughout our interviews and fieldnotes and are the norm for this group of families in which new mutations have led to new cases of haemophilia. However, even in these new families, sometimes 'a sharp-eyed nurse' or an 'on-to-it GP' brings about a speedy diagnosis, or an accident occurs and the family are in the right place to be diagnosed. This was the case for Luke, a little boy who was diagnosed in the early 1990s in Auckland city, when he was less than a year old. His knee had swollen up and a diagnosis of septic arthritis was being pursued. An arthroscopy was done, urgent blood tests carried out, and 'as soon as the results came through [the paediatric haematology specialist] came down and said we are taking you up to [the children's oncology and haematology ward], and [will] start treatment'. This whole process took less than 36 hours. Treatment turned out not to be blood products but a recombinant product that was just being registered as a medicine in New Zealand at the time. A supply had been gifted by the company that manufactured it. The parents knew about hepatitis C in blood products, hence their great relief when they learned that their product was to be a recombinant one and thus virus-free. Their boy would have a different experience of haemophilia than boys or girls born even a year earlier. In cases like this where diagnosis was speedy and clotting factor replacement therapy began quickly, the families were full of praise for the care they received. In all the situations outlined above the actors were Pākehā or, if more recently arrived, were native English speakers.

Other situations were more complex because of the family circumstances. For example, a family arrived in New Zealand from one of the Pacific Islands. In their home island the parents had realised that two of the children had some puzzling health problems and had visited local healers, with little success. After they arrived in New Zealand the children were diagnosed with haemophilia and had access to treatment from the health service. In another case, a family had adopted a baby who turned out to have haemophilia. This was not sporadic haemophilia because at least some members of the birth family were aware of the possibility of haemophilia, but this information had not been passed on in the adoption process, leading to a delay in diagnosis.

Some families know a diagnosis before the baby is born: approximately 70 per cent of babies with haemophilia are born to families with a known family history of this bleeding condition. Their experience is different from families with new mutations. In 'known' families, there may still be uncertainty about whether a child has a haemophilia mutation, but families know what haemophilia is, they know the level of severity in their family, and usually, but not always, new haemophilia is identified quickly. They may know from their prenatal care that the child about to be born is a boy or a girl. If the father is the parent with haemophilia and if the baby is a girl, then most people in this community know that the girl will be a carrier, and if the baby is a boy, that he will not be affected. However, if the mother is the person who has the haemophilia mutation, then a prenatal test is necessary if the parents want to know before the birth if their baby has inherited its mother's haemophilia mutation. Some women carrying haemophilia have prenatal testing to prepare themselves and their partner for the birth, while others may consider termination (see chapter 4).

In a minority of cases there is delay in diagnosis because of complications in the type(s) of haemophilia or because there are other things going on, such as von Willebrand disease. It may take many months for a complete diagnosis to be reached and this time of not knowing is very difficult for parents. This was the case for Nita, a parent in our 2006 update study. Her three-year-old son had not had a full diagnosis at that time, not because testing for haemophilia had been omitted but because achieving results proved very difficult (Park and York 2008, 9). The little boy first showed severe bleeding problems after an operation at around 11 months. Once he began toddling he began having joint bleeds and was tested again and found to have low factor VIII (FVIII) levels. The tests indicated that there appeared to be an additional mutation interrupting the clotting cascade. This was a very difficult diagnosis to make and our participant explained that so far, the geneticist had been working with DNA samples from about 15 family members. It had been five months since the samples were taken and her son was then more than three years old. On asking their families about their medical history, the parents of this little boy found that Nita's husband's mother knew that there was von Willebrand disease in his family, but she had not told them about it, even though she knew the baby was about to have an operation. Nita and her husband did not wish to have any more to do with his mother. However, Nita's family had no history of haemophilia, so the haemophilia mutation(s) was sporadic. Nita had found the diagnostic uncertainty upsetting and difficult to deal with, especially because it had not been possible to establish a routine treatment process, and she did not know what the future held for her son. The importance of 'putting a name to it', as Jutel (2011) titled her study of diagnosis, not just as a description of a condition, but as a prescription for action and a guide to the future is very evident in Nita's narrative. In this situation where something is clearly wrong, diagnosis would be a comfort. She expressed her sense of time stopping or slowing, while the uncertainty was prolonged.

NITA: He's looked after fairly well when he is in hospital, um, although with the diagnosis and tests and that, they just don't seem to have any idea of why he is like he is, which is really frustrating, because I can't sort of (sighs and pauses). It's hard, that side of it is really hard, because I need to know, if you like I need to be able to put him in a [diagnostic] box so I can understand exactly why and what to expect from him, but I can't do that yet.
JULIE: Yeah, so that is really, a lot of uncertainty there for you.
NITA: Very much so. I feel like my life has been put on hold until I really get him sorted and we work out exactly what is going on with him.

Becker (1997, 120), who studied how people narrated their experiences of disruptions in their lives, wrote that 'a period of limbo inevitably follows a life disruption'. Although talking about infertility, she found that the limbo metaphor applied to a range of illness or disability-related disruptions. She noted that uncertainties of the condition's progress or outcome exacerbated and prolonged the sense of liminality, of being betwixt and between, outside of, or slipping between, the normal structures of life. However, Becker arrived at the view that by using the limbo metaphor her participants were able, slowly and painfully, to begin the process of reordering their world, their identities and their futures. In this regard this sense of time out from 'life-as-usual' is comparable to the liminal periods of rites of passage where similar reorderings take place (Turner 1969).

This indeed seemed to describe the situation for Nita and her husband. Two years later when Julie met Nita again, her son had had his diagnosis for well over a year and their lives had settled into the routines of living with treatable, although complex, haemophilia and von Willebrand disease, starting school, sports, and so on. For them, life was on track once more.

For certain groups of people, receiving a diagnosis of haemophilia had particular effects on their sense of identity. A few women, especially in the first phase of our research, told us that they knew that haemophilia was a men's condition, so when their bleeding problems were attributed to haemophilia they were concerned about their sex/gender identity, felt very isolated, and worried about being able to have a family (see chapter 3).

As one woman said in 1995, 'I am different. I can't describe it, different to other women'. Another group for whom a diagnosis sometimes had specific identity effects was Māori. One woman told us that between when her son was diagnosed with haemophilia and her first visit to a Haemophilia Foundation camp where she met other Māori, she believed that her family was the only Māori family to have haemophilia. Thinking that haemophilia was a Pākehā disease, a not uncommon idea, she wondered about her family ancestry. She was very relieved to find that Māori seemed to have just as much haemophilia as anyone else, if not a bit more, possibly due to larger family sizes in recent generations. On the other hand, two Māori participants, or rather the families of two Māori participants, thought that haemophilia was the result of a Māori curse, which suggests that they accepted it as an indigenous condition, although this did not preclude biomedical explanations and treatments.

Medical condition or abuse

Gillian referred to the locum's suspicion of child abuse when her girl was covered in bruises, a common experience for parents of children with haemophilia. Parents received considerable attention from the public because their babies looked, as several parents described it, like 'bruised bananas'. Queuing at the supermarket checkout was a typical situation where this surveillance might occur with the bruised baby strapped into the trolley for all to see, but casual encounters on the street were not uncommon. This response occurred in all phases of our study and though it was unpleasant and upsetting for the parents, ultimately, they were pleased that the public and health workers were vigilant against child abuse. In several cases, it was this vigilance that led to diagnosis and effective treatment. Although, at the time, some of the mothers reported being angry at the looks they got from other people, the stigma of a suspicion of child abuse did not seem to affect the mothers' efforts to find out what was wrong with their child. They so strongly believed that 'something was not right', and they were so certain that it was serious, that they persisted, although realising, as one mother put it, that their doctor may have thought that 'I am a child beater'.

Tui told of a life-changing event with very serious health consequences for her son where abuse was suspected. Her undiagnosed baby boy became very ill with a brain injury and there was a serious delay while they were initially treated in a provincial hospital. Mother and baby were transferred to Starship hospital after a month. The police and social welfare were involved, Tui said, 'because we were Māori' and abuse was suspected. The eye specialist brought in to check for head injury actually saved the boy's life, according to Tui. He was able to rule out violence as the cause of cerebral bleeding, and the next most likely cause was haemophilia. A blood test taken soon after confirmed haemophilia, and treatment started immediately. The baby had extensive brain damage due to the month-long bleed into his brain but compensated well as he grew up. Tui's taken-for-granted association of the clinical suspicion of child abuse with her Māori identity was disturbing to her interviewer, Julie, and this association seemed to be implicated in the treatment delay: one month in a provincial hospital without adequate treatment. Although it was clear from many other stories that child abuse was suspected across all ethnic groups in sporadic cases of haemophilia, in this case, it was not so much suspected but assumed. To the shame of the New Zealand community, intentional injury of children is more common than haemophilia, and is therefore a more likely explanation for serious injury in children.[7]

Mild haemophilia

Another group who may have considerably delayed diagnosis and experience a different haemophilia are those with mild haemophilia. Although the clotting factor levels in this group are much lower than normal, often there are no serious effects in everyday life. A person might reach adulthood and only be diagnosed if a serious accident or surgical procedure results in excessive bleeding. Before DNA tests were available, the main diagnostic process was through clinical signs and a clotting time count. An older man explained in 1994 that he knew that he was 'a bleeder' from his family history and his experience of bruising and bleeding. He told the Navy examining officer this when he went for his medical. A clotting time test was duly done via a prick on the thumb and a stop watch. The diagnosis was, 'No, you are not a bleeder, you are in', so he joined the Navy. Later, however, he had some very serious health problems and new tests showed that he had haemophilia. Quite commonly, a diagnosis in their twenties allowed young men and women with mild haemophilia to explain some of their puzzling experiences, e.g., from a young man who played rugby all through school, 'So that's why I had all those bruises when I played rugby', or, from a keen sportswoman, 'That's why I am having some problems with my knees'. In these instances, the diagnosis provided a powerful 'Ah ha' moment. These experiences were retrospectively integrated into narratives of having haemophilia.

Although mild haemophilia was a serious health threat only under extraordinary circumstances, it had its own anxieties. Treatment for mild haemophilia is on demand rather than through regular infusions and families were therefore not as familiar with dealing with haemophilia as those who had to manage it daily. They usually did not have blood products at home, were not in close touch with regular treatment services or with the haemophilia community more generally and were not very experienced in deciding when a treatment was necessary. Paradoxically, our research showed that people with mild haemophilia had relatively high needs.

Caring for a child with haemophilia

Having a baby with haemophilia and being responsible for his or her care is a different experience of haemophilia than any other, especially for the first baby.

> Until they actually have their first bleed you don't actually know what you are looking for anyway... He was crying and we didn't know what was wrong with him.
>
> (Interview with parent in 1995)

The next day, the parents noticed that their toddler was drinking with his cup in his left hand. This observation of unusual left-handed drinking coupled with the baby not being happy led to the parents realising that he was having a bleed somewhere in his right arm or hand. It was not visible, but nonetheless detectable through various signs including touch. In this case, it was a serious elbow bleed whereas the parents had been concerned about a graze to his face.

Learning how to be vigilant is part of living with haemophilia as a new parent and continues over a lifetime. Much of the vigilance relies on sensory engagement, listening to whether a child is walking evenly, running hands over the child's arms or legs to see if joints are hot, which signals bleeding, and careful visual observation (Park 2013). Women who were familiar with haemophilia because of their experience with their brothers told us that even this close contact did not prepare them fully for parenting a child with haemophilia.

One of the emotions experienced by some parents is grief. A mother told us that after her son's diagnosis she cried for about a year. To console herself, she would go and look at him when he was asleep and remind herself that he was the same boy that he had been before the diagnosis. Her perfect newborn had been transformed into a child with a heritable medical condition by the act of diagnosis and she grieved for this present and future loss. A few fathers grieved for the loss of their imagined future rugby-playing star.

Where, as is most common, the child with haemophilia is a boy, the father's side of the family is unlikely to be familiar with the condition and what it means, because the boy has inherited haemophilia from his mother. If it is a girl, who may have inherited it from either her father or her mother, one or other side of the family will eventually have to start learning about haemophilia. However, unless the daughter is one of the 30 per cent of women carriers with low clotting factor levels, there is not the immediate anxiety about preventing, recognising, and dealing with bleeds, or making decisions about treatment.

In all phases of our research, many participants spoke warmly of the family support they received, and we could see this in action at haemophilia events and during our home visits. In the minority of cases where family support was not forthcoming, i.e., when a husband could not cope and left after the birth of a son with haemophilia, or went into a period of depression, or where the parents-in-law were critical and blamed the wife for bringing haemophilia into their family, the emotional toll was heavy. Sometimes the emotional toll was felt by grandparents, much like the grandmother 'time-bomb', where grandparents blamed themselves: they felt that it was their having a carrier daughter that had led to a grandson now suffering with haemophilia.

Families knowing a good deal about haemophilia through prior experience could be both positive and negative for parents. With improvements in the convenience and efficacy of treatment, a greater societal acceptance of and provision for difference, and safer treatment products, living with haemophilia in the twenty-first century is not the same as even 20 years ago, and is very different from 40 years earlier. For this reason, some of the fears of an earlier generation were no longer relevant for parents of young children or the teens and young adults. However, many participants told us that learning from the older generations about their coping strategies, their attitudes to life, and knowledge of health care was instructive for new parents or the newly diagnosed and a great source of support. Beyond the family, many stories showed how friends in the haemophilia community offered advice, support, and broader knowledge, and HFNZ and health services were usually necessary partners in the lives of families with newly diagnosed haemophilia.

He's a boy first: not living haemophilia

Although in this chapter we are concentrating on how people have described living with haemophilia, in fact in the lives of most of our participants, haemophilia is just one aspect. It is there alongside being a brother or mother, a schoolboy or university student, an electrician or lawyer, a grandparent, rugby fan, swimmer, musician, being Māori, Pākehā, or Samoan, living in Auckland or on a farm. Reminding themselves that their son was the same boy after his diagnosis as he had been before it, many parent-participants said to us something like 'He's a boy first'—i.e., his haemophilia is just one aspect of his personhood. For those who are office bearers in the Haemophilia Foundation or in the regional branches, haemophilia does occupy more of their lives, as it does for people who are seriously ill. But for the most part, as so many people said, their lives were 'pretty normal really' or they wanted to have or had had 'a normal life'. In fact, some parents said they 'didn't want to "live haemophilia"', but to get to a point where it occupied a small compartment of life, similar to the parents of children with asthma whom Trnka (2014) worked with. Living with haemophilia is, in the local idiom, 'Just getting on with it'. While this stoicism was expressed by older people in the community too, they had had a lot more to overcome to achieve this goal.

In a reflective interview with Kathryn in 1995, one older man with hae-mophilia, Robert, explained that when he felt a haemorrhage coming on it was not just the pain and the inconvenience that upset him but the pres-sure of associations going with it—'lots of disappointments and things'. Robert's individual experience of repetitive pain and memories of loss was widely shared and supports Cole's (2004, 99) argument that pain helps to produce memories. Men described in detail the types of disappointments that were remembered: missing the school concert, or sports day, or a family picnic, a holiday trip, one's own birthday, and even school exam-inations. In addition, with severe pain, relating to other people became problematic. Each new bleed had its own disruptions and pain and it called up a whole history of remembered and felt disappointments and pain that were part of the embodied experience of a bleed. Siblings of peo-ple with haemophilia often had to deal with the same disappointments of missing out, but not the bodily pain, although witnessing their brothers' pain could be traumatic.

Frequent severe pain in the absence of adequate treatment caused fre-quent recourse to pain relief, and concerns about narcotic addiction. We met men who had struggled with this themselves and grown-up children who had witnessed their fathers' predicaments. This was part of their expe-rience of haemophilia and part of what they brought to bear when, for example, evaluating the seriousness of haemophilia.

An older man who had struggled in this way found that when he was given control over his pain relief he was able to use much less medica-tion. This is a common finding in self-administered pain relief (see Hill *et al.* 1990). He reasoned that it was the fear of pain as well as the pain itself that had driven his high usage of pain relief. Once he could be con-fident that he could control his pain, that fear subsided. Unfortunately, in accord with changing ideas and technologies of pain relief, he was given this control only later in his life. By this time, he had been diag-nosed with HIV. In halting half-sentences he conveyed the suspicion and anxiety surrounding his dealings with some health professionals about pain relief and narcotics addiction in the context of his haemophilia and his HIV.

That these narratives are from older people is significant. Except for some people with inhibitors, prophylactic treatment or on-demand home treatment has almost eliminated repeated spontaneous bleeding for peo-ple with severe haemophilia by maintaining their levels of clotting factor in the moderate or mild range. It has allowed people in the severe and moderate ranges to take up pursuits that would have been impossible or highly dangerous before. Bleeds still occur but can be treated promptly and effectively so that the associations of pain and disappointment are not nearly so strong. Life has become more predictable and less painful for younger people with haemophilia and their families. Although improved treatment currently benefits older people with haemophilia, they embody the inadequate, or nil, treatment of the past in their damaged joints and the associated pain.

Having treatments

The goal of prophylaxis is to prevent spontaneous bleeds and to provide protection against bleeds from minor bumps and twists. This is accomplished by treating often enough and with sufficient amounts of clotting factor replacement that the trough levels are never too low. This goal is now easier to achieve than ever before. A single treatment for haemophilia used to take up to an hour, by the time the products were mixed and drawn up, the equipment readied, perhaps the area for the needle access numbed, good access to the vein secured, the transfusion itself completed, and pressure kept on the access point. With a fearful or grumpy child it could be longer. The details including batch number also had to be recorded and the treatment area kept sterile.

Although many of the elements are the same, products now are more ready to use, are more concentrated, and many folk thought that only five to 15 minutes were required. Trish described in 2006 how she no longer knows which mornings are treatment mornings for her teenage son, Ben, as he is so quick with it.

> We certainly noticed it, going from plasma-derived to recombinant products, because the recombinant, you're only taking a small amount, 10–15 mls, whereas prior to that we were doing 40–60 mls. You actually had to draw it up in several syringes and the whole giving, it took half an hour as opposed to the five minutes it takes now. Occasionally I'll say to Ben, 'When's treatment day this week?' Or 'When was the last time you had treatment?', and often he'll have had it that day and I just haven't noticed, it was sort of so quick. But he is very independent with it now.

This is the end-point of a learning process. First parents, then boys and the occasional girl must learn these techniques and perfect them. Many mothers and a few fathers talked about their fears when they themselves were learning, describing good days and bad days, but most became competent in the end, sometimes after a period of complete loss of confidence. A few found another relative, such as grandmother or grandfather, to give the treatments or relied on a nearby clinic. One mother, for example, did not want her child to associate her with the discomfort of treatment, so the boy's grandmother did treatments.

Learning how to do home treatment was a milestone for many parents, especially mothers. Intravenous injections are not easy, even for health professionals. For some mothers, like the one below interviewed in 1994, the impetus came from having to stand by while her son was given injections by a whole range of different doctors. As she and several other mothers said, they knew their son's body very well:

> [At first] I didn't have the stomach. I'd seen the needle put in so many times by the doctors and then I realised that each time I went to a doctor, he'd get a new one [a different doctor]. I probably knew [my son's] veins better and I knew the child and it was probably easier... if I practised I wasn't going to be a lot worse than some of the doctors.

Other families lived rurally, including Ursula, introduced earlier in the chapter. She had had to steel herself to learn to give injections.

> Well, I was needle phobic, so it was horrendous for me. Now it's fine. Initially I used to have heart palpitations and it was just a nightmare. I hated it really and I hated it because initially I wasn't very good, and sometimes we didn't hit the vein and it would be unpleasant. Now it's pretty well one go, and so it's not [too unpleasant].

Similar views were expressed by the 13 Swedish carrier mothers of boys with haemophilia in Myrin-Westesson, Baghaei, and Friberg's (2013, 222) study. Becoming skilful in giving intravenous injections to their children demonstrated a 'turning point' in their journey as mothers of boys with haemophilia.

Another turning point is when the boy himself starts helping with the process and eventually takes it over (see Figure 2.1). Tui and her son lived rurally and had another stay at Starship in Auckland when her son had

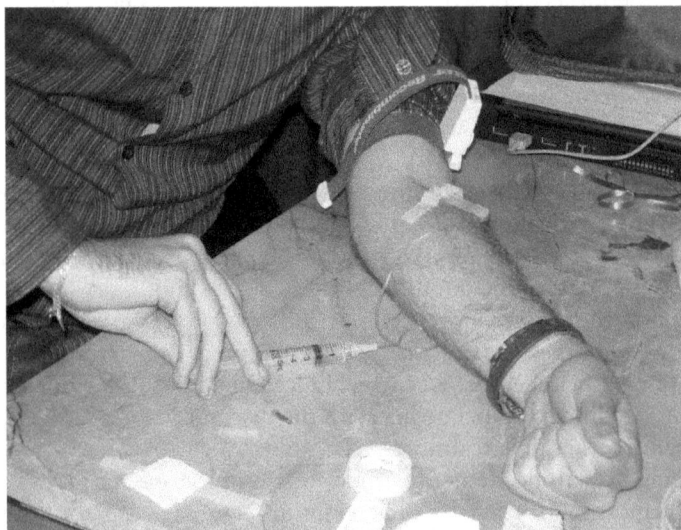

Figure 2.1 Infusion of clotting factor replacement.

his portacath inserted. She spent one day with the nurses there practicing infusing clotting factor on the dummy patient, and then, she said, 'We more or less taught ourselves after that'. She had help from the nurses at her local hospital a couple of times who gave her lessons on transfusion, and then it was up to her. 'My mum and myself used to do it. My mum used to hold him down when he was a baby and I used to do it'. But now he helps get all the equipment ready and Tui does the infusion herself. She is looking forward to the time when her son can take it over. But building up parental skill and developing cooperation in the child is by no means a linear process, as Ivy, whom we introduce shortly, discovered in what was quite a common process of two steps forward and one step back.

In some areas of New Zealand, small children usually have portacaths inserted. This is to avoid the repeated need for venous access, to make infusion easier, and to preserve the child's veins. There are some regional differences in the use of portacaths as they can get infected and need to be removed, replaced, and the infection treated, and their insertion is a surgical operation. Some haematologists advised parents to begin direct intravenous access at the beginning of home treatment, as scary as that was. These two different approaches were the cause of much debate among parents. The children with portacaths (called 'ports') seemed to accept them well. For example, on one visit to a country home, the little boy ran out to greet Julie as she pulled up in her car. He asked her what she was going to talk about, his mother having primed him. When Julie said, 'About haemophilia', he flipped up his T-shirt to show his portacath and said, 'I have haemophilia'. Another little boy had drawn a self-portrait that showed three little circles on his chest. He explained that one was his portacath, the others were his nipples. Some adults may also use ports, for example if all the usual veins have collapsed.

The episode below was about a little boy and his parents changing from using his portacath to administer treatment, to direct access to a vein.

IVY: It was awful. ... it started off quite good, I don't know, he was really good for a start off, 'cause we started off doing it twice a week in his port and once in his arm, sort of thing, and then we went twice in his arm and once in his port, and then we weaned him right off and were just doing the port once a month, because we had to flush it, he was quite good, but once his port was actually gone, he sort of changed. And, I don't know. Maybe, they said, maybe he thinks his safety net has gone, and he was really naughty, I don't know if you would say naughty, screaming, yelling, kicking. It was awful.

JULIE: It must have been pretty tough.

IVY: We started going to the hospital again, which isn't very far to go [in their own town], it didn't really matter. Then they [nursing staff] started coming out at home, then they started me doing it at home again and slowly got him back, and me building up my confidence again, you know.

Other parents described how at different times they or their partner either lost their confidence after one or two difficult infusions or became a *persona non grata* to the child for a while and the other parent had to step in. As children became older they would start to take part in the process, for example by helping to get the equipment ready, like Tui's son. At haemophilia camps or sometimes in clinics, or at home if there were an older brother with haemophilia, they might see an older child giving himself a treatment. In fact, it was common at family camps or boys' camps to see the older boys infusing themselves in the treatment room and several younger boys watching with various degrees of hero worship. Eventually children with haemophilia would learn all parts of the process, including the scary bit of inserting the needle into a vein. This is routine for a child with haemophilia, not something exceptional. Being able to infuse yourself was a mark of growing up—not exactly a rite of passage, but definitely a cause for congratulations and pride. But for children, too, it was not always a simple progress toward perfecting their technique. Sometimes the parents or health professionals would have to take the task back—perhaps due to a loss of confidence, an outbreak of the grumps, or a bleed in the operative hand or elbow that made manipulating the equipment very difficult.

Becoming skilled at home treatment as a parent or a child is part of the self-management of haemophilia. It takes its place along with vigilance, first aid expertise, calculating risks and benefits from taking part in activities, e.g., maybe rugby is too rough, but soccer is better, or soccer is too risky, but archery is OK; keeping careful track of the amount of product used, when treatments and bleeds occur, and making adjustments to timing or amounts; making sure the car always has petrol in it in case of emergencies, and keeping the cell phone charged. With just a couple of exceptions of people with moderate or mild haemophilia who preferred to attend the GP or hospital for treatments, after the initial scary period, home treatment was experienced as a great convenience. But convenience was only part of the story. It was necessary to prevent bleeding episodes as it enabled regular, frequent, prophylactic treatment and promptly administered extra treatments in the event of day-to-day trauma. Despite the time it took and how it turned a small part of the house into a temporary sterile area, it enabled life to be 'pretty normal'. Home treatment, in conjunction with long-term relationships forged with regular doctors and nurses and the mutual support and shared expertise found within the haemophilia community, enabled the development of parent-experts and patient-experts.

After years of home treatment, parents hope that their adult children will be able to look after themselves when they leave home. Albie, a young man who had been living independently for several years, is an example of this realised hope. He talked about his active approach to staying healthy, including regulating the quantity and frequency of his treatment, as well as his exercise routines and other aspects of daily living. He was on prophylaxis for severe haemophilia.

ALBIE: I do about 1000 units every second day, and that's a high dose now. I'm on a much higher dose now than when I was young. I recently, about two years ago, looked at the CSL ... recommendations for my weight, and I was on far too low for a severe haemophilia so I upped the dose as they suggested and it's been good. See, then I was doing more less [frequently], now I'm doing less more. So really, what I am doing is trying keep that sine curve [graph of the up and down of the clotting factor levels in his blood] from going too low, too high, so there's going to be smooth.

JULIE: Every two days is quite often, so how do you find it fits in with everything else you have to do?

ALBIE: See the whole thing with it is, it's the beginning of a normal life: treatment. Without it, my life isn't so normal. It's ah, I think I put up with it more when I was younger, the bleeding and the pain. I don't have as much time for it now, I think that is where, as you get older, you don't have as much time for a lot of nuisances (laughs) ... Mum's not there, Dad's not there. I have to be more able—to put it simply, so that means, look after yourself and prevent any possibilities you have to knock yourself back.

Like the New Zealand parents of children with asthma, described by Trnka and McLauchlan (2012), parents of children with haemophilia, and men like Albie, saw pharmaceuticals as key to maintaining normality. Like the 'asthma parents', parents and adult patients also did some tinkering with the home treatment regimen, such as giving an extra treatment before sports, or having more frequent, lower dose treatments. Sometimes this was discussed with their doctor, but sometimes done on their own initiative. But unlike the asthma parents, parents and people with haemophilia did mobilise in collective action around national treatment standards. There are several reasons why this difference might be so, such as the relative rarity of haemophilia compared with the frequency of asthma, the inter-generational nature of the condition, and especially the collective mobilisation around the blood-borne infections. Although parents and patients take responsibility for home treatment of haemophilia, and in this sense they have been made to be responsible (Rose 2006), this collective mobilisation to devise national standards of care demonstrated that people with haemophilia believed that responsibility for care was shared with the State. They combine active and social citizenship. The State was responsible not just for safe treatment, but for provision of good quality treatment across New Zealand and for ensuring equity of access (see chapter 6).

Blood-borne infections

Treatment with blood products exposed people with haemophilia and other recipients of blood and blood products to hepatitis B and C and to

HIV infection. Because haemophilia treatment is repeated over many years, some men got all three infections, with hepatitis B being noted as a 'side effect' from midcentury until blood was screened for it after the virus was identified in 1967. HIV infection scarred the 1980s until adequate tests and screening methods were discovered, and hepatitis C (though probably present in the blood supply all along) was a particular feature of the late 1980s and early 1990s when at last the virus was identified, tests became available, and effective treatment of blood products instituted. By early 1993, it had been eliminated from the products used in New Zealand.

Although blood products have never been safer and recombinant products are not implicated in these diseases, many people still expressed concerns about safety even in our 2005–6 restudy. These were not at the pitch of the fears expressed in 1994–5 or 1999. Creutzfeldt-Jakob disease, other hepatitises, and a general fear of TNV (the next virus) were mentioned. As one mother described it in 2005, 'I'm 99.99 per cent sure that we will never receive anything [treatment product] that is dodgy, but there is still that 0.01 per cent that says, "Oh, I hope that's OK"'. Unusually for a toddler, her son was on a plasma-derived product because of treatment difficulties with synthetic products. A father whose son was on a recombinant product always made sure he got this and not a plasma-derived product if they had an emergency and were not having home treatment. This was partly because of safety fears, even though he 'knew' that the plasma-derived product was just as safe. Knowledge alone was not sufficient reassurance for him to allow his son to have it. We took this well-educated man's approach as an indication of how deeply scarred the community was and noted how that scarring was not confined to the pre-1993 generation.

Inhibitors

Haemophilia treatment has made a world of difference to many people with haemophilia and to their parents, but clotting factor replacement therapy is not successful for a percentage of people, variously estimated as up to 20 or even 30 per cent. This is because they have developed inhibitors. Instead of the replacement clotting factor lasting within their bodies according to its normal half-life and helping clots form, it is attacked as foreign material and destroyed quickly. Inhibitors occur with both blood products and recombinant products and the process is not yet fully understood. For treatment in these cases a different factor to the missing one is used. This enhances clotting but is not usually as effective as if the actual missing factor were able to be used. In recent years, a process known as tolerisation is used, usually with small boys, because the amount of product used in tolerisation, as in treatment generally, is dependent on body weight (Paisley et al. 2003). The plan is to give the child so much specially formulated treatment product that their inhibitors will be overcome, rather like having lots of bee stings can reduce one's reaction to stings. If successful, as it usually is, then the child can subsequently be treated with the correct clotting factor in the usual way. A fear of developing inhibitors from a different product prevents some people with haemophilia or their parents from changing their treatment products, e.g., from blood-derived to recombinant, or to different brands of recombinant product. Like the severity of haemophilia, a tendency to inhibitor development also seems to run in families.

In New Zealand, prophylactic treatment is not usually given to toddlers, partly to observe how their haemophilia is expressed and partly in the hope of reducing the numbers of children with inhibitors. Parents found this period when treatment was only on demand, during which time children took lots of tumbles and knocks, very difficult, as they would have to work out when treatments were necessary and were of course worried about trauma without the reassurance of the higher clotting factor levels obtained through prophylaxis. Thus, even people without inhibitors were affected by this attempt to avoid them.

Having inhibitors can present problems if other health issues come along. For example, an older man with a FVIII deficiency who had developed a FVIII inhibitor but was quite well-treated by factor IX for everyday life, told us in 1995 that he was advised by his haematologist not to have surgery for another medical problem because there might be difficulties in controlling bleeding. If inhibitors develop, the surgical operation of putting in a portacath becomes more difficult because large amounts of the relevant treatment products have to be amassed to ensure that bleeding can be controlled.

Parents as liaison officers

Setting children on the path of self-treatment and teaching them how to deal with the various complications that haemophilia brings is a key part of parenting a child with haemophilia. But it is by no means the end of this particular journey. Once children move out of the family context there is a great deal more work to be done. Parents then become what we have termed 'liaison officers'.

Because haemophilia is a rare condition, most people in the general community know little about it. Typical 'knowledge' might include that it used to be in European royal families, it is a royal disease, it had something to do with the Russian revolution, and people with haemophilia can cut themselves and bleed to death (Berger 1989; Resnik 1999). Consequently, parents, caregivers, and children themselves have substantial work to do to educate and reassure people with whom children with haemophilia will be spending time. This includes educating about invisible bleeds, creating a supportive but not restrictive environment, and what to do when accidents inevitably happen. Many parents joked that their children had inherited 'the monkey gene' along with a haemophilia one. By this they meant that the kids were very active, climbed anything, ran everywhere, and generally tended to push limits and terrify their parents.

Each time a child with haemophilia undertook new activities with new people, parents and caregivers acted in a liaison role, often assisted by materials provided by HFNZ, phone calls from outreach workers or sometimes health care professionals, such as the haemophilia centre or a GP. Operating on a need-to-know basis, the parent would inform relevant adults and sometimes the child's close friends, about haemophilia, about their boy or girl's needs regarding safety, and who to call for help. Cell phones have allowed parents, especially mothers, freedom and peace of mind, knowing that the preschool, school, sports coach, and other parents can contact them at any time in an instant provided they are within an area with cell phone coverage.

The choice of preschool and school loomed large in many parents' minds, especially in the early years of our research. The behaviour of other children and the attitudes of staff were keenly observed. If they did not feel that the school could keep their child safe while enabling him or her to participate, and respond appropriately to emergencies, parents would move their child elsewhere.

One mother in the 1995 study described the look of relief on the face of the kindergarten teacher when she arrived to collect her son at the end of the session.

> ... some people are frightened of haemophiliacs. The kindergarten was probably the worst. The head teacher at kindergarten wanted him to have a helmet and all sorts of things. ... She tells me to this day that she still was scared stiff that he would hurt himself.

In 1994–5, many children had not been getting adequate treatment by today's standards and families had to make complex decisions around school attendance. Consistency in schooling can help avoid problems of isolation and stigmatisation, but some young people felt more comfortable at home rather than going to school when they had obvious mobility problems, and this too could avoid stigmatisation. The parents of the boy described in the next excerpt had decided that keeping his school attendance regular was the main issue.

> I always maintained that if I could get him upright I could get him to school. So we had crutches here, and once again he fought for normality too, so he wouldn't use crutches unless he really had to. I had two or three slings that I put different transfers [attractive pictures] on for him. ... As far as the schooling goes, he's got to be basically dying and in the ambulance before he doesn't go to school. We cart the wheelchair, we cart the crutches, he parks up in the beanbag.

But sometimes going to school with visible mobility problems draws unwanted attention.

...what we are trying to achieve... is to keep his days off school to a bare minimum... [5–6 days] have been because he had an ankle bleed and it's just too painful for him to get around the school because he doesn't like to have the haemophilia drawn to attention.

(Mother of 14-year-old with severe haemophilia in 1995)

Neither of these excerpts would be part of the experience of children in our more recent studies, except in case of exceptional accidents or uncontrolled inhibitors.

Some parents were apprehensive that school would be the site where their boy would learn he was different. Ursula's son, Uri, was about to start school in 2006.

He isn't aware that he is different from other children at the moment, because he isn't different. It will only be when he goes to school and can't do the contact sports, I think, that he will really know, so I'm not looking forward to it.

Note that it was sports, rather than school itself, that presented the potential problem for Ursula. Sport does present a challenge in the New Zealand context, despite many clever parental strategies.

An adult reflecting on his schooling many years before had had a good experience of school sports:

The school was actually very good. The first day they said to me, 'If you want to play rugby, you go out and play rugby, it's yours to deal with'... So that freedom was very important, so was the lack of control that they were trying to exert over me in terms of, 'Oh you've got a condition, we want you to stay in a corner'.

(Man with severe haemophilia who chose not to play rugby)

Other adults had not been so lucky and had been made to play rugby because rugby had been compulsory at their school. Alternatively, the teachers were so terrified that the boys had been prevented from taking part in what would have been reasonably safe activities. Such rigidities have largely disappeared from the educational scene, with the increase in the number of sports on offer and with teachers who are better educated in inclusive education and can relate to and provide for children with a wide range of disabilities or illnesses. Even so, parents' stories suggest that sometimes a little extra thought and flexibility would allow students with haemophilia to participate even more, for example in school trips, school camps, and other outings. This was another context in which different haemophilias were evident (see Benseman and Park 1998).

Some teachers may still be wary of children with haemophilia, but more recent parental accounts suggest that this is relatively unusual. Prophylactic treatment has removed more of the scariness, and treatment improvements also meant that by 2006 most children lost very few days of schooling, and could safely participate in a wider range of activities. However, some of the credit for change must go to the inclusive environments provided by many schools, the policies and practices relating to safety, and efforts made to foster responsible relationships between children.

At all phases of the study children, parents and teachers were inventive in strategies for inclusion.

> [The school] let him do what he wants to do, and when they are having running races, like at the end of the year, he helps set the course out, he keeps an eye on the kids or whatever. The teachers give him a job so he's not left out.
>
> (Mother of 9-year-old)

But the children can be sensitive to these special efforts as they grow older:

> His teacher pushed him around the cross-country course [in a wheel-chair]. And another mother offered to dress him up as a rally driver with a crash helmet and push him around this year. But he was a bit sensitive about it at that stage and he said no, he'd rather not.
>
> (Mother of 6-year-old)

Making a child stay behind while the rest of the class went on an outing was fortunately not commonly reported. The issue of school camps and trips involving children with haemophilia caused consternation in some schools. Parents could find themselves caught between the school that wanted them along and the son for whom having mum or dad along was the last thing he wanted: 'The shame!'

Reactions to the blood-borne viruses, which hit the headlines from 1984, created difficult environments in some schools, as a man who had been at secondary school at the time explained.

> When I was at school, AIDS came on the scene. A lot of haemophiliacs had it, and I remember my brother was given a hiding by some other guys at school because they thought he had AIDS. And as a consequence I think it's probably why he buries his head in the sand about his condition.

These two brothers had moderate haemophilia: one had treatment and enjoyed the support of the haemophilia community and the other tried to ignore his condition. This is a vivid example of the health effects of bullying. A few parents described having to go to great lengths to convince schools that teachers and other students would not get infected by AIDS from children with haemophilia.

While there was considerably less hysteria about hepatitis C, some people chose not to tell the school that the child had the virus or chose schools where hysteria was less likely. One father reported that if his son with hae-mophilia had a 'bleed at school, no one wanted to touch him because they knew he had hep C'. However, this did appear to be rather exceptional. Post HIV, most schools had clear protocols for safely dealing with blood.

Children with haemophilia, with the help of their siblings and parents, are also active agents in their education, developing strategies that give them satisfying educational experiences and enable participation in a wide but selected range of school activities. The following family conversations were part of our 1995 study, but were replicated in all phases.

KATHRYN: Have you found it difficult to explain to your friends why you are not doing rugby or anything?

SCHOOLBOY: No, I just say I've got haemophilia and I can't do it because I can't risk hurting myself.

MOTHER: They are a really nice bunch of kids here. Some of his friends are really lovely, understanding...

JULIE: Do your friends at school know that you've got haemophilia?

SCHOOLBOY: Yeah, most of them do... just my friends.

JULIE: Do you think they treat you differently?

SCHOOLBOY: No. Oh they do if I do something that will hurt me, they tell me to be careful or whatever.

JULIE, JOKING: They are your conscience?

MOTHER, LAUGHING: Someone has to be!

These different experiences were part of the different haemophilias created through a combination of the way the boy or girl with haemophilia han-dled the condition, the school's approach, the treatment available, parental attitudes, and the biological expression of an individual's haemophilia.

Adults working and living with haemophilia

Education is highly valued in this community and is linked with obtaining employment compatible with having a bleeding disorder. Parents, talking about their son in 1995 said:

> Obviously he shouldn't go into manual labour or things like that, so he really does need a good education, and he needs to have some sort of tertiary education to get him into white-collar jobs. And that's a big fear that I have, because he really has to be better than the next person to get the job.

In 2006, a young man in his 20s discussing his education and employment strategies, given that he had haemophilia and hepatitis C, used almost the same words: 'I have to be a little bit better than the next guy'. He used this phrase to explain that to have an 'equal' chance at a job, he had to be better than the field, because his medical conditions would place him behind the starting line. One of the pleasures of doing this research has been meeting up with the young adults whom we first met as children, who are now engaged in a wide range of meaningful enterprises, and have completed or are completing their tertiary education. Within the haemophilia community are chefs, sport coaches, lawyers, teachers, architects, scientists, hairdressers, administrators, salespeople, a sprinkling of skilled tradespeople, and even an anthropologist.

The HFNZ has a specific fund devoted to providing grants to assist members to access the education they need to provide satisfying lives for themselves and to broaden their opportunities for employment compatible with having haemophilia. It is difficult to over-emphasise the importance of education in this community.

The narratives of adults with haemophilia make very clear the difference that home treatment and prophylaxis has made to work, education, and life in general, especially for those with severe and moderate haemophilia. Accessible building design for people with walking problems has also been a plus. One 1995 participant who wanted to undertake a job as a rugby administrator was prevented by the office being in a block with no lift or disabled access and by the international travel required. These days, even with severe haemophilia, building access and travel difficulties are only exceptional problems, although travel takes considerable organisation.

Older men pointed out that before there was adequate treatment for haemophilia, it was possible to get a job because there were more jobs than there were people to do them: a situation not replicated in the last few decades. However, promotion often passed men with haemophilia by because without good treatment, they were classed as unreliable. This meant that they remained on lower wages or salaries during their working life. Once in employment, men found that the key was to have some flexibility. Even so, work cycles and the wish not to let workmates or the boss down led a number to work when they should not have, thereby exacerbating bleeds or other health problems. With more effective and safer treatment, this is not such an issue, but it has not disappeared. Prophylactic treatment is designed to stop spontaneous bleeds and to limit the damage from other bleeds. It does not prevent all bleeds. Men may still have to get up at 2 a.m. to have a treatment if they feel a bleed coming on, despite prophylaxis. But for the last two decades, they have not been at risk from HIV or hepatitis C.

More men with severe levels of haemophilia thought that their employment opportunities had been 'quite a bit' or 'severely' affected by the condition. These reported restrictions included not being able to be in the army or police force, although one man with mild haemophilia was a police officer, or not taking jobs requiring frequent international travel or too much mobility, and some other jobs that were too risky. However, we did meet a butcher and a glazier, neither with severe haemophilia, and one young man is an award-winning chef.

There are many continuities regarding work over the three phases of our research and the remembered time beforehand: the approach of the employer is key. Being flexible, allowing a person to 'make-up' time, and providing physically safe working conditions for people with 'dodgy' joints were consistently important, although the need for flexibility has reduced somewhat with better treatment. From 1995, a middle-aged man said:

> They were good to me. I suspect they thought I was a reasonable employee. And when I was no longer able to write [because of damage from repeated elbow, wrist, and finger joint bleeds] they gave me a different position where I didn't have to write.

Several of the men's narratives from this time use the phrase 'good to me'; and allude to a sense of reciprocity. The understatement of 'a reasonable employee' could be rephrased as a very valued staff member who had worked hard and well. In return, the employer found suitable work for him, or, in other men's stories, carried on his wage while he was sick, or transferred him from an hourly wage to a salary. Invariably, the employee made up the time when the crisis was over. In a few cases, however, the narrators thought the arrangement veered toward exploitation: 'he expected his pound of flesh [and that I would work all hours to make up for time off]'. And some employers were not inclined or not able to employ a person who was frequently off work or unable to perform certain tasks.

The men's strategies around employment are also key. In all age groups, but particularly in the over-40s, a larger proportion of men with haemophilia, compared with the population at large, were self-employed and others employed a small staff. Based on our discussions with them and sometimes their wives, we interpreted this as a further strategy to increase flexibility (Park *et al.* 1995). Men with haemophilia who were employers generally had a right-hand man or woman who could carry on if they had to have some time off work, and as several pointed out, only this way could they run a viable business. A man in his 30s with severe haemophilia said in 1995 that he became self-employed as soon as he had finished his apprenticeship: 'No one else would put up with the time I have to have off. But on the other hand, you can't ring in and say you are not coming and you don't get any sick pay'. Having one or more trustworthy employees made running a business more feasible. One older man told us when we visited his company workplace in 1995:

> The young fellow out the back, he's very good, but he knows damn well if I lift anything, he's seen what happens if I do. Now he says, 'Leave it boss', and he goes bloody crook [tells me off] if he sees me lifting anything.

Others have taken stock when their work was proving difficult and tried another tack. Albie, who was introduced earlier and took part in the 2006 study, described how he had qualified and worked in a job he enjoyed very much, but which had entailed having to carry around a lot of heavy gear. He later realised the amount of treatment product he had been getting was too low, and his lifestyle had not been healthful and he had been careless. As a result, he had experienced repeated bleeds. He developed target joints and was not always able to do his job. At a certain stage of his life when things were going badly he took charge of his treatment, changed his lifestyle to one which he thought was healthier, and negotiated a desk job in the same industry. This meant he could do his work even if he was having bleeding or joint problems. His work was not as satisfying, but he had developed other interests about which he was passionate.

There were other barriers to achieving the goals that many New Zealanders aspired to. For example, because of difficulty or extra expense in gaining life insurance, more than 60 per cent of men with haemophilia had either been refused it, or had not applied when we enquired about this in our 1994 survey. We were told that the extra loading on the premium could be 200 per cent. As having life insurance was formerly a requirement for some home mortgages, men who wished to buy a house had to devise strategies to overcome this barrier and to provide for their dependents.

An 'overseas experience', or 'OE', is seeing the world by spending time overseas often building up international experience in a career, and is a rite of passage for many young New Zealanders. One middle-aged man told us in 1994, 'Before the concentrates came out [in the 1960s] I would never have dreamt of going overseas. It would have been too difficult'. Depending on the destination country, travel often involves organising the supply of replacement factor and medical referrals. Even after the 1960s, travel was not easy because concentrate needed to be refrigerated and was bulky and heavy. Customs officers could create problems over the syringes and medical kit, even when medical documentation was supplied. People who were unable to self-treat were often concerned about accessing good treatment overseas. On the other hand, the desire to travel was sometimes a stimulus to learn the intravenous transfusion procedure.

> I got somebody to take a photograph of me after I put my first needle in, beaming smile on my face. From then on it was a different world. I had it [treatment] on sailing boats in the Hauraki Gulf, I had it at Nambasa rock concerts in the back of a van.
> (Man who learned to self-treat as an adult, talking in 1994)

For those with joint damage, mobility was a problem, and HIV status also proved an issue for entry to some countries. The greater transportability of treatment products and much more widespread use of self-treatment have assisted Kiwis with haemophilia to fly, although they still encounter a few hassles along the way. As in so many other areas of life, the resources of the World Federation of Hemophilia and several member countries have made travel easier with travel advice and lists of haemophilia treatment centres.

Haemophilia and getting older

Each person's experience of treatment for haemophilia is different. Some people in their middle years and older find that they need much less in the way of treatment products and can reduce their intake with no ill-effects. The current treatment guidelines suggest that prophylaxis will not be needed past early adulthood and instead treatment on demand will suffice, but this seems to be very flexible in practice and many adults were having prophylaxis. Adults, usually with clinical guidance, experiment with the effects of treatment on demand versus prophylaxis and with the amount of treatment product per infusion and frequency of treatment to come up with the most economical and clinically best treatment that works for them. We were often regaled with the record keeping of men who experimented with a variety of treatment modes before settling on their current treatment regimen. The current cohorts of mature men and some young adults who for a variety of reasons—inhibitors, lack of product in their region, lack of access to good care—did not have adequate treatment when they were younger, often have painful joints and require treatment for arthritis caused by their haemophilia. Joint operations to restore mobility and reduce pain are common, as are visits to the physiotherapist. Of course, many of these men and some women also had the effects of hepatitis C and required the intervention of gastroenterologists. There is a keenly felt thinning in the ranks of the haemophilia community because of deaths due to HIV and hepatitis C.

Having a whole cohort of older men with severe haemophilia is a new phenomenon, enabled by the availability of safe and effective treatment products and good health services and self-care. This particular experience of mature people with haemophilia will not be repeated as the current young people and young adults grow older. Although some of those who were born before 1993 have not been able to clear their hepatitis C, or only cleared it in 2016, and some relatively young men did not get adequate treatment or had untreated inhibitors and so do have damaged joints, for most younger people, severely damaged joints, viral infection, and intense on-going pain relating to haemophilia is not going to be their experience. These different haemophilias have the potential to create some tensions within the haemophilia community as successive cohorts have different needs. With so much necessary attention in past years being devoted to the youngsters, their parents, the younger adults, and the people with the blood-borne viruses, the older people recently have voiced their needs as the first generation who are aging with haemophilia. In response, a new 'masters group' of these senior men has been created within the Haemophilia Foundation and they have had opportunities to get together and discuss the challenges and responses in their lives. In the Wellington region, for example, a group of 'masters' meet frequently to do physiotherapy exercises. This is unknown territory as it is only since the latter part of the twentieth century that almost all men with severe and moderate haemophilia can expect to live to old age. Elliot (2016) explored some of the issues for older men in New Zealand, as did our study 20 years earlier (Park *et al.* 1995, 144ff.), and found that mobility issues and their implications for independence and physical activity, the complexity of dealing with having haemophilia and other health problems, and concerns about the cost of haemophilia treatment and its implications for them were all important issues. There are many questions yet to be asked and answered about how having haemophilia interacts with the local biology of aging in New Zealand.

Conclusion: local biology and different haemophilias

Our research suggests that generation, age, gender, place of residence, ethnicity, and changing treatment circumstances are some of the most important considerations in creating different haemophilias. These important differences along with national or cultural backgrounds, socioeconomic circumstances, family history, social context, and quality of general health care, interact with the biology of the specific genetic mutation to create a local biology of haemophilia in Aotearoa New Zealand. Local biology highlights the ways in which social, cultural, and biological processes are entangled over time to produce human health and illness (Lock and Nguyen 2010, 90). Personal characteristics including psychological dispositions, spirituality, worldview, ethical orientations, sexuality, understandings of the condition, and even body-build are also part of the processes that create different haemophilias. Haemophilia is also different depending on whether one is a doctor, a geneticist, a person with haemophilia, or their parent or sibling. For one person, it is just a bleeding nuisance, for another, it is devastating, and for another it is a medical condition for which she has a passion.

As Mol (2002) theorised for arthrosclerosis, these different haemophilias are also the same haemophilia, united particularly by health care records and the practice of diagnosis. Although haemophilia A and B require different clotting factor replacements and are genetically different, haemophilia is treated in similar ways, is diagnosed by genetic and haematological experts, people with it are cared for by the same network of specialists, and served by the same Haemophilia Foundation. People with haemophilia of a certain age have been exposed to the same dangers through contaminated blood products, they have struggled together to get adequate treatment, and all age groups risk the same problem joints and mobility issues. Haemophilia is both single and multiple. As we discuss in the next chapter, the differences are not fixed. The changing status of women as 'expressed carriers' to 'women with haemophilia' is but one example of this.

Many areas of life, such as family relations, leisure activities, and people's interest and passions do not figure in this chapter. Some of these topics are threaded through or more fully developed in the following chapters and we hope our readers will gain glimpses of the warmth, humour, and challenges of family life, and more rounded views of the lives and personalities of people with haemophilia.

Notes

1. Older people with haemophilia often refer to themselves as 'haemophiliacs' or 'bleeders'; many people refer to themselves or others as 'a haemophilia', and most people recognise the phrase 'people with haemophilia', which we use as a respectful reference.
2. Although haemophilia A and B are single gene disorders, the specific mutation, such as a deletion, a replication, or an inversion, is likely to influence the expression of haemophilia in each instance.
3. Predicament is a concept borrowed from Shakespeare (2008). It invokes an active response and works well with the concept of local biology, as it does not privilege the biological.
4. All names of research participants are pseudonyms.
5. Plunket nurses provide free well child services to children younger than five years.
6. Bleeds into the brain or the central nervous system are extremely dangerous.
7. An average of 24.3 hospitalisations per 100,000 for boys for intentional injury between 2006–10 (NZCYES 2011).

References

Becker, G. 1997. *Disrupted Lives: How People Create Meaning in a Chaotic World.* Berkeley: California University Press.

Benseman J, and J. Park. 1998. 'A Bleeding Nuisance: The Implications of Haemophilia for Education'. *Australasian Journal of Special Education* 21 (2):81–97.

Berger, M. 1989. *Understanding Haemophilia: A Personal Account and Practical Guide for Parents, Teachers and Caring Professionals.* Bath: Ashgrove Press.

Bönisch-Brednich, B. 2002. *Keeping a Low Profile: An Oral History of German Immigration to New Zealand.* Wellington: Victoria University Press.

Buchbinder, M., and S. Timmermans. 2011. 'Medical Technologies and the Dream of the Perfect Newborn'. *Medical Anthropology* 30 (1):56–80.

CDC. 2015. 'New Study Findings: Research Study Shows that Female Hemophilia Carriers Have Evidence of Joint Abnormalities'. http://www.fwgbd.org/news/new-study-findings-research-shows-female-hemophilia-carriers-have-evidence-of-joint-abnormalities (accessed 11 Nov, 2018).

Cole, J. 2004. 'Painful Memories: Ritual, and the Transformation of Community Trauma'. *Culture, Medicine and Psychiatry* 28:87–105.

Elliot, S. 2016. 'Explorations into the Unique Issues and Challenges Facing Older Men with Haemophilia'. Master of Social Work Thesis, University of Auckland.

Garro, L.G., and C. Mattingly. 2000. 'Narrative as Construct and Construction'. In *Narrative and the Cultural Construction of Illness and Healing*, edited by C. Mattingly and L.G. Garro, 1–49. Berkeley: University of California Press.

Good. B., and M.J. Del Vecchio Good. 1994. 'In the Subjunctive Mode: Epilepsy Narratives in Turkey'. *Social Science and Medicine* 38 (6):835–42.

Hemophilia Federation of India. 2014. 'Welcome to HFI'. http://www.hemophilia.in (last accessed 11 Nov, 2018).

Hill, H.F., C.R. Chapman, J.A. Kornell, K.M. Sullivan, L.C. Saeger, and C. Benedetti. 1990. 'Self-Administration of Morphine in Bone Marrow Transplant Patients Reduces Drug Requirement'. *Pain* 40 (2):121–29.

Jutel, A.G. 2011. *Putting a Name to it: Diagnosis in Contemporary Society.* Baltimore: Johns Hopkins University Press.

Kleinman, A. 1988. *The Illness Narratives: Suffering, Healing and the Human Condition*. New York: Basic Books.

Lock, M., and V-K. Nguyen. 2010. *An Anthropology of Biomedicine*. Malden, M.A.: Wiley-Blackwell.

Mol, A. 2002. *The Body Multiple: Ontology in Medical Practice*. Durham: Duke University Press.

Myrin-Westesson, L., F. Baghaei, and F. Friberg. 2013. 'The Experience of Being a Female Carrier of Haemophilia and the Mother of a Haemophilic Child'. *Haemophilia* 19:219–24.

NZCYES. 2011. *The Children's Social Health Monitor 2011 Update*. Dunedin: New Zealand Child and Youth Epidemiology Service. http://www.nzchildren.co.nz/index.php.

Paisley, S., J. Wight, E. Currie, and C. Knight. 2003. 'The Management of Inhibitors in Haemophilia A: Introduction and Systematic Review of Current Practice'. *Haemophilia* 9 (4):405–17.

Park, J. 2013. 'Painful Exclusion: Hepatitis C in the New Zealand Haemophilia Community'. In *Senses and Citizenships: Embodying Political Life*, edited by S. Trnka, C. Dureau, and J. Park, 221–41. New York: Routledge.

Park, J., and D. York. 2008. *The Social Ecology of New Technologies and Haemophilia in New Zealand: 'A Bleeding Nuisance' Revisited*. RAL 8. Department of Anthropology, The University of Auckland. https://researchspace.auckland.ac.nz/handle/2292/4534 (last accessed 11 Nov, 2018).

Park, J., K. Scott, J. Benseman, and E. Berry. 1995. *A Bleeding Nuisance: Living with Haemophilia in Aotearoa New Zealand*. Department of Anthropology, University of Auckland.

Phadke, S. 2011. 'Hemophilia Care in India: A Review of Experience from a Tertiary Centre in Uttar Pradesh, India'. *Indian Journal of Hematology and Blood Transfusion* 27:121.

Resnik, S. 1999. *Blood Saga: Hemophilia, AIDS, and the Survival of a Community*. Berkeley: University of California Press.

Rose, N. 2006. *The Politics of Life Itself: Biomedicine, Power, and Subjectivity in the Twenty-First Century*. Princeton, NJ: Princeton University Press.

Shakespeare, T. 2008. 'Disability: Suffering, Social Oppression, or Complex Predicament'. In *The Contingent Nature of Life: Bioethics and Limits of Human Existence*, edited by M. Düwell, C. Rehmann-Sutter, and D. Mieth, 235–46. New York: Springer.

Thayer, Z.M., and A.L. Non. 2015. 'Anthropology Meets Epigenetics: Current and Future Directions'. *American Anthropologist* 117 (4)722–35. doi:10.1111/aman.12351.

Trnka, S. 2014. 'Domestic Experiments: Familial Regimes of Coping with Childhood Asthma in New Zealand'. *Medical Anthropology* 33 (6):546–60.

———. 2017. *One Blue Child: Asthma, Responsibility, and the Politics of Global Health*. Stanford, CA: Stanford University Press.

Trnka, S., and L. McLauchlan. 2012. 'Becoming "Half A Doctor": Parent-Experts and the Normalisation of Childhood Asthma in Aotearoa/New Zealand'. *SITES (NS)* 9 (2):3–22.

Turner, V. 1969. *The Ritual Process*. Ithaca, NY: Cornell University Press.

3 Blood and sacrifice

Sex, gender, and haemophilia

> But for him to pick one sport that he really wants to do, for it to be rugby! It could have been anything you know.
>
> (Ivy, the mother of a 'rugby mad' [her description] little boy talking to Julie in 2005)

'But it couldn't have been anything', Julie thought, 'it *had* to be rugby'. She asked Ivy more about rugby in her family and in their rural community. Ivy explained that her husband used to play rugby when he was a boy, and 'he watches all the rugby on the television'. 'Watches *all* the rugby?', Julie mused to herself, 'that would be a lot!'. As Ivy described it, rugby is built into the social fabric of her district, as it is throughout New Zealand. Each winter at their local school, all the girls play netball and all the boys play rugby. Their school team is part of a district competition, an essential building block of interdistrict sociability and social networking, as de Jong (1987) demonstrated in his historical study in Taranaki. Ivy's son's district plays other districts, their provincial area competes with others, and so on, continuing up to the All Blacks, the national team. This feature of rugby social organisation has been evident in New Zealand for over a century (de Jong 1987; Fougere 1989) and ties New Zealand to a national and international circuit of sporting relationships, building a key feature of masculine and national identity up from the grass roots. Rugby and other key sports enact gender, sexuality, and class and speak to intergenerational ties, ethnicity, and nationhood (Lewis and Winder 2007; Park 2000; Phillips 1987; Pringle 2002).

Gender is a key component of local biologies of haemophilia. We explore how the X-chromosome-linked, 'sex-linked', genetic condition of haemophilia is also and always a gendered experience. Following Bourdieu, especially in later works such as *Masculine Domination* (2002), we theorise gender as an embodied disposition, part of habitus, which, borrowing from Mol (2002), is enacted. 'Enacted', in Mol's sense, is not intended to convey self-conscious awareness but to suggest that phenomena such as gender or haemophilia or arthrosclerosis are continuously created, re-created, and modified through everyday practices. These practices may be as varied as record-keeping, laboratory analysis, home treatment, clinical encounters, the distribution of pharmaceuticals, or playing sport. In this respect, Mol's concept is comparable to Butler's 'performativity' (1990), but enactment, as these examples suggests, is multifaceted and moves some distance from the discursive, speech-act, basis of Butler's performativity. Enactment is field- or context-related and sometimes open to strategic deployment, but it is not entirely free as it encounters the sediments of past enactments, such as embodied and external gendered structures, or medical hierarchies.

Embodied gendered structures are evident in, for example, Ivy's son's 'choice' of rugby, while external structures are the nationwide arrangements for competition and the connection of high achievement in sports to fame and fortune. These structures are not unchanging or unchangeable, but often change only as a result of considerable struggle. We exploit these theoretical concepts to examine how dominant gender structures and values have shaped men's and women's embodiment and enactments of haemophilia, concealing some dimensions of haemophilia, while emphasising others, and how this has changed over time. We attempt to indicate how gender interacts with these other dimensions, creating complex patterns of and for haemophilia. In doing so we echo the scholarly and societal reworking of gender in a rethinking of health studies as a gendered domain.

The history of health studies has been marked by the exclusion or invisiblisation of women. Kaufert (1999), for example, reviewed the famous 'Whitehall' studies in public health[1] that were key to putting social inequality and stress as a health hazard on the map. Yet the first Whitehall study included no women and the second, she convincingly argued, did not see the different story told by the women's data because of the epidemiological cultural practice of data aggregation and 'adjusting' for sex (or gender), which obliterates difference. Kaufert (1999, 125) wrote, 'In their own way, these analytic techniques are as effective as is the *chador* in concealing the female presence. Everyone knows she is there, but by being veiled she becomes invisible'. In the case of haemophilia, women as people with it are invisibilised not just through social and academic processes, but also through the biological and genetic characteristics of the condition, which mean that few women have severe haemophilia.

The significance of genetic sex in the haemophilia community revolves around the unique consequence, in terms of blood's ability to form a clot, of having one or two X chromosomes. Males with haemophilia have one affected X and one Y chromosome so are not protected against mutations on the X chromosome. Females, having two X chromosomes, have a good chance of being protected when they have one affected X chromosome because haemophilia is a recessive mutation.[2] But sex in terms of X and Y chromosomes is not the same as sex in the sense of sexuality, nor is it the same as gender. Local constructions of gender interact with the sexed biology of haemophilia, sexuality and other social and cultural dimensions, and health service provision to create different Aotearoa New Zealand hae-mophilias. We use a plural here because both haemophilia and gender are affected by many other things, giving rise to a multiplicity of understand-ings, experiences, and enactments. We intend, with this and the follow-ing chapters, to provide further insights into local biology and different haemophilias.

In New Zealand haemophilia, bleeding men have been the focus of atten-tion, as one would expect given the major health and mobility issues they face. But as potential fathers and carriers of a haemophilia mutation that they pass on to all their daughters, they have been neglected (Park 2000, 451). While some men had always known that they would transmit haemophilia, very few paid it much attention. In our research we found several men who believed that they could not pass it on, and swore that their doctors had told them this.[3] Others learned about men's role in transmitting haemo-philia only later in life.

In contrast, women as people who bleed had been almost ignored or even denied until very recently, whereas their sacrifices as mothers, wives and caregivers and their status as carriers were widely acknowledged in the haemophilia community (Park 2005). As researchers we were no differ-ent in our approach when we began our study. We had been so convinced by our reading and discussions of the rarity of women's bleeding due to haemophilia that we were amazed that nine women (out of nearly 200 respondents) completed our questionnaire as people with haemophilia, although several of them did this tentatively, writing 'they didn't know if they should'. By the end of this study we, and most other people in the com-munity, were aware that approximately one-third of women with a haemo-philia mutation have reduced levels of clotting factors, such that many of them experience symptoms of mild haemophilia and a minority have more severe bleeding issues, as discussed in chapter 2. We explore these findings and relate them to gender in New Zealand society, especially examining how masculinity has coalesced around rugby and sport in general, how femininity has revolved around reproductive issues, and how these associa-tions have been challenged and changed in recent years.

The absence from the record of women as people with haemophilia can partly be explained by the likelihood that they will have mild or perhaps no symptoms at all. However, following Kaufert (1999), we suggest that more is at stake here. That women are now publicly acknowledged as hav-ing haemophilia-related bleeding disorders, for example on haemophilia websites in New Zealand, the United States, and elsewhere, whereas 10 or 15 years ago, they were not, is not due to a sudden outbreak of women's bleeding problems. Rather, it is due to a change in recognition, brought about through a lot of talk and work mainly by people in haemophilia com-munities worldwide. The gendering of haemophilia provides a vivid illus-tration of anthropologist, Douglas's (1970, 65), observation so many years ago: 'the social body constrains the way the physical body is perceived'.

How this happens is why we turn to theorists like Mol and Bourdieu. Data collection and medical writing about haemophilia embodies the values and beliefs of those who do the work, just as this book does.

We tell the stories of masculine haemophilia in the first part of the chapter, and about the recognition of women's haemophilia in the second part of this chapter. We hold our main discussion of 'having children' until chapter 4. We begin by discussing the famous (in New Zealand) game of rugby as a key symbol of masculinity.

Rugby: a key symbol

Ivy's community is rugby focussed. In 2005, Ivy reported people commiserating with her and her husband about their son's haemophilia by saying 'I don't know how I could handle it if my son couldn't play rugby!' We heard similar remarks from other rural towns elsewhere in New Zealand during all phases of our research. However, Ivy described herself and her husband as unaffected by this social pressure. She said that they think 'Well, so? It's not the end of the world!'

Perhaps there is a slight change here exemplified by Ivy describing her family as 'unaffected' by the social expectations that focussed on rugby in comparison with the views of the father in another family with haemophilia interviewed in 1995. We were speaking about leisure activities. Both parents and the boy in question were present. The mother suggested that 'touch rugby', a form of the sport with little body contact, was a 'good compromise'. The father disagreed saying that 'the worst hassle' about haemophilia, 'is you can't play rugby', while their son backed up his dad, agreeing that not being able to play was 'stink' (Park 2000, 445).

However, the difference between these two families may not be entirely due to change over time. Rather, it is possible that Ivy unwittingly de-emphasised the importance of rugby to the men in her family as did her counterpart in 1995. This tendency for the boys' mothers to deny the importance of rugby was the case in other conversations in which both men and women participated. For example, Art, a father in another rural area spoke in 2005 about all the sports that his seven-year-old son was doing, including swimming. He described his son's distress when the time came to register for rugby, and how as a dad, he came to realise what a 'big deal' it was for his boy not to be able to play.

> Art: I knew it was a big deal when that triathlon happened ... [My son] did the swimming length for his team and got them well up in the places from what they were and the others were saying, 'Good swim!' to him and he suddenly went from being on this lower plane of not being able to do that stuff [i.e., play rugby] to being (gestures: a hero), so he was back 'in' with all the boys. 'I don't have to play rugby cos I am back in', sort of thing.

Art's account points to the importance of sport for social relationships among the boys: for being 'in', being accepted. The lesson Art drew is that rugby is best, but winning or performing well in another sport 'for the team' can *compensate* for not playing rugby. During this conversation, the mother's brief contributions had been to diminish and de-emphasise the pervasiveness of rugby, e.g., 'He's not the only one who doesn't play', perhaps trying to make it 'all right' that her son could not play, in an example of maternal 'emotion work' in which the well-being of relationships and those within them is the goal (Hochschild 1979). However, the family conversation that ensued revealed that the only other boy who did not play in this age grade had a health problem.

These examples are all rural ones; unsurprising given the rural connections of rugby (MacDonald 1996; McCaw with McGee 2012; Philips 1987). Rugby as an inevitable presence was almost universal among rural families—whether they loved it or not—however the presence of rugby was by no means confined to them. Many of the city-dwelling adult men whom we got to know talked to us about rugby. It was important for many, but not all, of them. If they could not play it, they could consume it in other ways, by being knowledgeable about it, by reading about it, by watching it, by loving it, or by helping to organise it (see Figure 3.1). The rural-urban difference is one of emphasis rather than a qualitative difference: rugby and the allegedly rural values of stoicism, perseverance, and mateship which it often invokes are important to ideas of nationhood and masculinity in New Zealand for rural and urban dwellers alike (Belich and Wevers 2008, 6; Phillips 1987).

One example, this time about a city boy, shows that it is not just the lack of choice that causes boys to turn to rugby. It also demonstrates again the difference between the mother's and her son's views. In her interview, the mother of this 11-year-old (in 1994) described three different sporting activities that her son was doing, including rifle-shooting, which he was good at and enthusiastic about. She felt that he was a lot happier and more settled having found something he could fit in to. But unknown to her, her son wrote 'plaintively and privately in his questionnaire response, "I would love to play rugby"' (Park 2000, 445), making us feel sad when we read it, both for him, not being able to realise his wish, and for his mother, who had gone to such great lengths to create a rich and engaging environment for him. These other sports also allow boys to embody force and competence, which Connell (1987) identifies as key components of masculinity central to sport, but our work suggests that in many cases other sports are *substitutes* for rugby.

The centrality of sports and rugby to relationships between New Zealand fathers and sons is no doubt a powerful channel for creating the sense of regret expressed by men and boys. A few fathers of sons with haemophilia spoke of this, and so did some men with haemophilia in relation to their own inability to keep up with their son's play as their boys grew

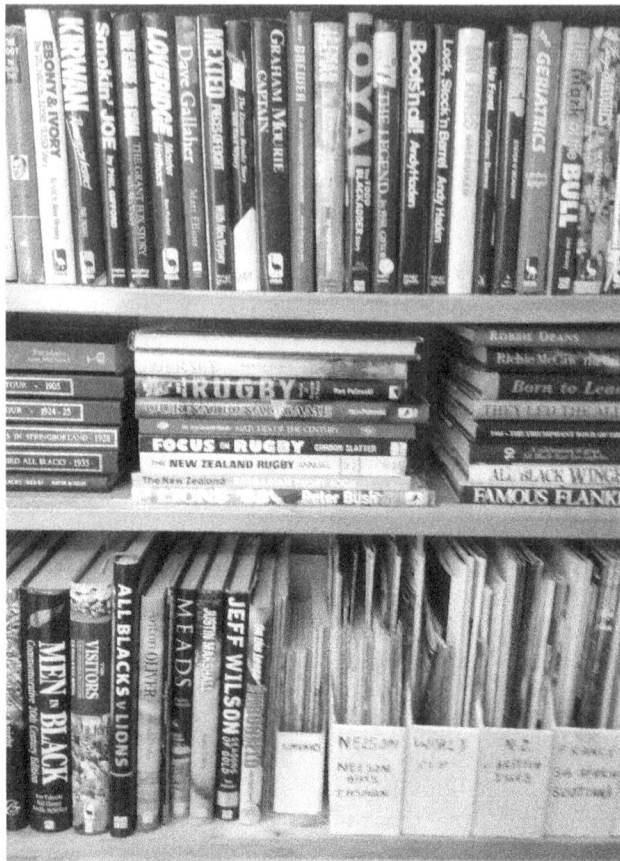

Figure 3.1 A participant's library of rugby books.

older. However, the most powerful sense of this cross-generational regret came from wives and mothers who reported how disappointed and even depressed their husbands had been when they found out their sons had haemophilia and could not play. In a few extreme cases, this had been the last straw and the marriage had dissolved. In a few other instances, it was the key symbol of loss associated with their husband's depression (Park 2000).

Despite the greater ranges of sporting and nonsporting activities on offer in the twenty-first compared with the twentieth century, rugby is still the game of New Zealand. In the build-up to a Bledisloe Cup rugby test match between the Australian Wallabies and the All Blacks in August 2008, the Auckland newspaper (*New Zealand Herald*, 31 July 2008, A1), which has a large urban readership, invited readers to write in their 50 words of coachlike advice, and asked some rugby greats to contribute. Two columnists also wrote longer articles in a similar vein. The results were published over the next two days (August 1–2, 2008) in the main news section of the paper, not the sports section. Among the phrases used were:

'The jersey you are wearing was awarded to you by 3,999,999 Kiwis. Do them proud',
  'A team of 15 in our hallowed black',
  'We are all relying on you, but most of all you are relying on each other',
  'Your country is suffering in the grip of a fierce winter of despair. They look to you for hope and inspiration, because you are an All Black',
  'You're a team, you're New Zealand –YOU ARE ALL BLACKS!'
  Columnist, Jim Hopkins concluded his piece: 'Because that's who you are tonight. A team *and* a country. You win, we win. It doesn't make sense, but possess it anyway ... you are who we are'.

Even dissenting voices inevitably acknowledged the importance of the game by saying in their efforts to play down its importance, or to support their team:

'It's just a game',
'If you lose that's fine',

These readers obviously felt it was an important enough event to warrant writing a brief letter to the paper, as did 300 others over that two-day period (*New Zealand Herald*, August 4 2008, A1).

This game was played at a time when the country was being lashed by severe storms in which lives were lost and multimillions of dollars of damage incurred. At the same time, economic gloom and doom consequent on the ripples from the global economic crisis and the high price of oil were widespread. To cap off all this gloom, and perhaps worst of all, the All Blacks had lost badly to the Aussies in their previous game. But on that night at Eden Park, the All Blacks won by a large margin (39-10), cheering up much of the citizenry for a while. Three years later, again after a very difficult time for the nation—Canterbury earthquakes, a mining disaster with the loss of 29 lives, devastating storms and floods—the six weeks of the Rugby world cup of 2011 and its madcap supporters brought distraction and relief to the imagined 'stadium of four million'. It seemed that most of the population engaged and the mood lightened.

In our haemophilia research, even people who were not followers of rugby and who provided many alternative activities for their sons found themselves confronted by the importance of rugby and related sports in their communities. One Māori family had returned to their rural tūranga-waewae ('home area') after some years overseas. They resisted the assumption that rugby was the foundation of the meaning of life and contested local gendered structures. The mother explained that she was against rugby because of the image it created for men, because of the roughness and injury, 'even without haemophilia' and the associated drinking. She thought 'Society has to change how they are bringing up their men, their boys'. Her husband agreed, critiquing the

> 'whole macho scene. My extended family was really into playing rugby league.... Just being at the marae [Māori ritual and community centre] sometimes and they'll say, "Oh, when's your boy going to play, what team's he going to play for?" It was just assumed that all boys would play'. (Park 2000, 451)

This couple, like Ivy, also reported that people sympathised with them when they explained that their boys could not play because of haemophilia.

Rugby has been described as a national obsession, religion, or a barometer of the nation's health (Ryan 2005). No difference was detected between Māori and Pākehā in the interest in rugby or rugby league, nor were differences detectable on the basis of class. In Aotearoa New Zealand, rugby is a relatively egalitarian sport. While the version of Rugby known as League is a more working-class game, Rugby Union 'Rugby', attracts players and supporters from all classes (Palenski 2015).

Haemophilia social and business meetings were frequently enlivened by rugby talk and rugby jokes. Living 'a normal life', with taken-for-granted heterosexuality, was also often expressed in terms of rugby: 'I've lived a normal life. I played rugby in my youth' (man with mild haemophilia), or alternatively, rugby is part of a remembered diagnosis of haemophilia and an indicator of something wrong: 'Your son has haemophilia and will never play rugby' (doctor breaking the diagnosis of their newborn's severe haemophilia to the parents). Men who were not followers of rugby often mentioned this 'failing' in humorous terms, such as a young man who was into water sports who whispered in high irony to Julie (when only he and she were present) during an interview in 2005, 'I've never followed rugby.' Rugby and related contact sports are cultural facts of life over which both men and women stumble.

Rugby is part of the experience of haemophilia, and how New Zealand men and women enact their gendered identities. It has all the features of a key symbol (Ortner 1973). It acts as a gendered idiom of normality in the haemophilia community and in wider society. Like the flag, the national anthem, the silver fern and the haka, with which rugby is associated, rugby can stand for the nation or for 'normal masculinity'. But rugby also lays out a correct mode of being—hard work, determination, participation, coping with pain, loyalty, looking after your mates, and striving to be the best that you and the team can be—and sets up gender relations that stress a passive supportive role for women. However, as shown by the reactions of some families with haemophilia, through the increasing importance of women's rugby and touch rugby, which is a noncontact unisex sport, the advent of gay rugby, as well as the increasing popularity of football (usually called soccer in New Zealand), both rugby and its ordering processes are constantly being renegotiated and resisted. As a component of national identity and community spirit, it operates as a moral device for some New Zealanders. This is seen very clearly in advertising that draws on rugby imagery. But not all New Zealanders are believers. As Desmarais (2004) indicates, the images advertised are often in contradiction to the actions of rugby players. For example, while some All Blacks lend their support to campaigns against domestic violence, others are convicted of assaulting wives or partners.

Sport in general is a point of tension within the haemophilia community. Many of the most loved sports are on the 'Don't Play' list (Joll 2005), which no doubt only enhances their attractiveness. Boys and young men often confessed that they had concealed the extent of their sporting activities from their parents—mothers were particularly mentioned—but were 'outed' when they sustained an injury that led to a bleed. As adults, several men felt the effects of their early enthusiasm for sport, coping with damaged ankles and knees due to inadequately treated or repeated bleeds into joints. Parents faced the conflict between 'wrapping their child in cotton wool' (a metaphor repeated at all phases of the research that speaks of 'sissiness' and 'overprotection'), and 'allowing him to be a *boy*' and run, climb and play as much like other boys as possible. A strategy many parents pursued, noted in an earlier example, was to enrol their son(s) who were keen on sports in a game that did not have such damaging consequences as rugby or rugby league. However, some families got caught out when their sons turned out to be very talented players in these other codes and continued playing right up through the grades, thus exposing themselves to the possibility of on-field crashes with now much heavier and faster opponents, for example on the soccer field. Trade-offs between health, fitness, self-esteem, and sociability versus the possibility of injury, and use of extra treatment product before games were very much on the minds of these parents and their teenage boys. It was not too different for some adults who chose sports, such as surfing, where an accident could have serious consequences, but where the everyday exercise it provided and the enjoyment and focus it brought to life made it a valued pursuit. 'I just love it' or 'It's his passion', conveyed to us the meaningfulness of sports to some of our participants.

These teenage boys and sporting adults did not lie about their activities to their haemophilia doctors or nurses but nor were they very explicit. One adult regretted that his haematologist did not seem to appreciate that his favourite water sport allowed him to live a much healthier, happier life that in turn enabled him to limit his bleeds and cope with his haemophilia more effectively. Haematologists with whom we have spoken and HFNZ are very aware of the benefits of sport and social participation and the cultural importance of this to men in New Zealand. However, like everyone else in the haemophilia community, they are also aware of the personal costs when accidents happen, including delayed personal costs of damaged joints, and financial costs in terms of clotting factor replacement products and other health services, which they have a responsibility to use effectively and fairly. Our observations suggested they trod a fine line in this difficult area.

Over the years of our research, we noted greater parental confidence in introducing children into sports and greater knowledge of the increasing range of sports available in many, particularly urban, places. This is a result of the greater availability of prophylactic treatment and, some in the community think, of the promotion of sports involvement in this community by pharmaceutical companies that consequently benefit from increased sales of their products. More effective treatment for many of the boys with inhibitors also means that more of them can participate. HFNZ has also done a good deal of work on sports and recreation, for example, schemes to reduce the costs to parents of children's participation in safe sports, through talks and by example at camps where children are exposed to sports from angling to kayaking to rock-climbing, encouragement from outreach workers and physiotherapists, and through *Bloodline* and more informal contacts (see Figure 3.2). As a result, the next story, told in 1994 by the mother of a young urban teenager with severe haemophilia, is already (almost) a thing of the past.

> And he doesn't play any sport. He's already got [damage to his arms and legs and he limps]. All that sort of thing at this age group, he hates it because it draws attention to the fact that he's different from the rest and he just wants to be treated like the rest, but he can't be. So, socially, that's a real downer because he doesn't participate in anything on Saturdays with the rest of the school kids, like sport, so he hasn't got a social group to go out with. This year I've noticed this more than any other time of his life. … He's always left out.

Striving to have 'a normal life'

Taking part in sporting activities with other people was an important aspect of what many men with haemophilia called 'living a normal life'. It was an important, and indeed, the most talked of aspect of social participation—but not the only one. Yet the orientations and values discussed in terms of the key symbol of rugby can be detected in these other endeavours. As we discussed in chapter 2, getting an education that would allow men with haemophilia to pursue a career that will not exacerbate bleeding episodes loomed large, initially for parents and later for their young adult sons (Benseman and Park 1998). Although lonely weeks or months of enforced bed rest was no longer the experience of young boys and men, except for those with uncontrolled inhibitors, the sense of needing to strive more than

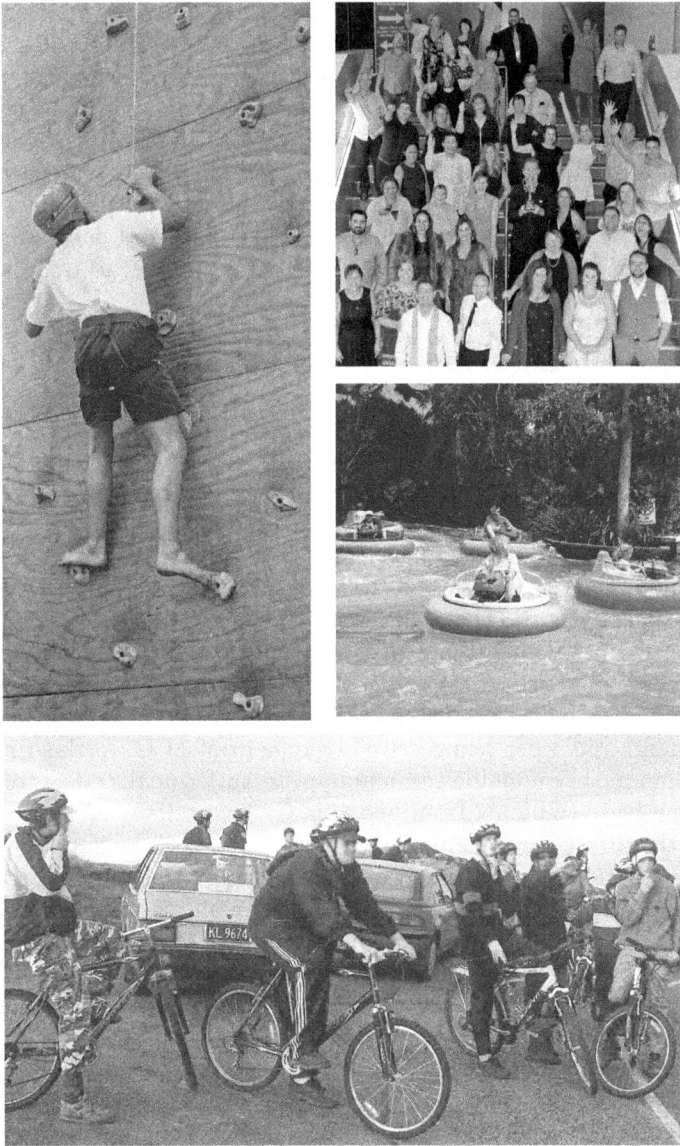

Figure 3.2 Community activities.

'the next person' was expressed at all phases of our research. Several young men talked about how haemophilia had made them more determined:

> I had my own group of friends. I worked hard to get to the top of the class. I guess I had to prove myself in other ways. I worked really hard to make up for that little bit of stigma that was attached.

The emphasis on education and training, and the determination expressed in the excerpt above paid off for many of the adults. In the next excerpt about work, 'a bit more determination' is an enormous understatement. This determination is part of the enactment of haemophilia, being inculcated from a young age as the children learn to live full lives with their haemophilia, and it is modelled by young and older men. The participant had just told us that when he was a little boy, his doctor told him he would never have a full-time job. He did have a full time and demanding professional job, he told us that he knew he would not get to the top of his profession, but that he had a lot to be proud of.

> I've got to work twice as hard as the next guy. I can say, 'I'm under pressure today, so is the next guy, but at least he didn't have to get up at 2am to give himself a treatment'. In some respects it has given me a bit more determination.
>
> (Man with severe haemophilia and virus infections,
> in 1995 when he was in his early thirties)

This striving that we argue is part of the enactment of masculinity symbolised by rugby, was similarly reflected in the employment statistics of our participants. In our initial study, when general male unemployment was 7.2 per cent (Statistics New Zealand 1996), only 1 per cent of the working age participants were unemployed, 12 per cent were on sickness and invalids' benefits and 4 per cent received income from ACC. At this time, several men in the haemophilia community were suffering the effects of AIDS, and some had symptoms from hepatitis C. These illnesses were in addition to the direct complications of haemophilia, such as damaged joints. Educational success was also reflected in the types of jobs that the men had, with more than 50 per cent being in professional, management or skilled trades, and more than 40 per cent in clerical, sales, and semi-skilled jobs. Being an economically productive and contributing member of family and society was a key goal for a very large number of people with haemophilia. It sometimes took a mighty effort, and often required careful strategising.

Paid work was not the only arena in which men strove to contribute as citizens. Men whose condition meant that it was not feasible for them to work, and others who were in paid work, devoted many hours to various forms of voluntary work. This included work within the haemophilia community and related activities, as well as a wide range of other services such as on the board of trustees for their children's schools, sporting administration, and various charitable associations. While these men could not be part of a rugby team, they participated in group activities in other ways. Identifying and striving to overcome obstacles to living 'a normal life' was part of living with haemophilia.

When we unpacked the content of the concept of 'a normal life' through our discussions with people with haemophilia and sometimes with their parents, we discovered that the goals and values summed up in the key symbol of rugby are to be found in these other areas of life. Creating a meaningful life through work, play, family, and other social relationships, striving to do ones best (or better), and generally participating in society in a wide range of ways are all part of the package. In more personal terms, rugby as a key symbol directs attention to men with haemophilia as people who bleed, lead active lives, need treatments, struggle and overcome their difficulties, or are tragically overcome by them. In the rugby imaginary, despite women's rugby, women are more often the behind-the-scenes workers and supporters: women make sacrifices so that men can play (and bleed). This is part of the work that rugby does in contributing to the way masculinity and femininity are enacted in New Zealand. Simultaneously, these gendered practices contribute to the local biology of haemophilia. Quite simply, if rugby and related contact sports were not so important in New Zealand, the experience of men and boys with haemophilia would be different: different yearnings and disappointments, different patterns of bumps and bruises, different experiences of social participation and exclusion. More complexly, the gendered relations and ideals of citizenship that rugby symbolises also work to produce local enactments of haemophilia epitomised in practices from rugby jokes as a mode of friendship to women's 'carrying'.

As a condition that affects men more severely and dramatically than it affects women, haemophilia slides neatly into New Zealand gender structures. However, this fit is neither exact nor static: there are loose ends. In the next section, we explore how femininity is enacted within the haemophilia community and analyse struggle and resistance in this enactment. Finally, we come back to some neglected aspects of masculinity.

Women in the haemophilia community: carriers and carers

'Carrying' and 'caring' were the ways in which femininity was publicly enacted in the haemophilia community when our research began. Women with haemophilia mutations were referred to as 'carriers', as in the phrase 'men with haemophilia and women carriers'. In our research, we have attended to the way stories we tell are powerful in bringing our worlds into being (Lupton 1994). This common phrase 'and women carriers' created a common-sense world in which men with haemophilia do not carry it and women do not have haemophilia. In medical terminology, if women bruised or had other bleeding issues this was not because they had haemophilia but because they were 'expressed' or 'symptomatic' carriers. They were usually attached to the haemophilia community by their kinship link to the men with haemophilia in their lives, the men they cared about and cared for: they were Max's mother, William's wife, Don's daughter and Sam's sister (Park 2005).

'Carry' can subsume both caring and carrying. If women are haemophilia 'carriers', they have a mutation for haemophilia on a particular gene on an

X chromosome, and some may even carry guilt about this. Whether or not they carry this mutation, as New Zealand women, they carry a responsibility of care for their relatives, including husbands, brothers, fathers, children, and grandchildren, who do have haemophilia. They carry the weight of bringing the next generation into the world. They carry the baby. With changes in available technology, women now more than ever also carry the main burden of decision-making about the use of technologies, which can help them limit the numbers of children with haemophilia.

Caring: 'I haven't been to medical school for seven years'

Women usually do the bulk of childcare in New Zealand, as elsewhere, even in two-parent families (Jones 2008, 10). Although many fathers are heavily involved in the care of their children with haemophilia, and some families alternate which parent gives home treatment, mothers are the lead caregiver in many families and sometimes the sole caregiver. Lucky parents also get help from their own parents, usually the mother's mother, but sometimes grandpa helps too, and sometimes the father's parents.

A child's diagnosis and bleeding impacts everyone in the family, but frequently the mother had to deal initially with the first bleed of her son, or occasionally, her daughter. One mother whose baby's diagnosis had not been confirmed at the time of her first interview with us in 1995, spoke of the horror she experienced: all that red blood on a white pillowcase.

> And I'll never forget going and picking him up out of bed. His pillow was saturated with blood. He wasn't bleeding when I put him to bed. I rang the GP and he rang me straight back and I took him to A&E [Accident and Emergency Department of the hospital].

Such bleeds, which are usually the result of teething, are terribly shocking, especially in families like this one where there was no inkling that the child had haemophilia. Fortunately, this slow bleeding from the mouth is usually picked up quite quickly and is not life threatening, despite its ghastly appearance. A diagnosis of haemophilia, a treatable condition, can come as a relief at such a time. But from then on, mothers and some fathers take on a range of quasi-medical roles. Not only will most of them learn how to do intravenous injections, and to judge when extra treatments are necessary, but they also learn how to manage their child's care.

Women can experience these caring responsibilities as quite a burden, wanting to do the best to prevent their child being damaged, but not being resourced to do so confidently. This was the case for Marie, a mother we encountered in 1994:

> It [care and responsibility] seems to have been all handed over to me. Which is good in a way, but I haven't been to medical school for seven

years! I don't know the whole background. And often things don't get done unless I initiate it. Like his ankle should have been picked up ages ago ... Then finally, after years of this, someone suddenly said, 'We will refer on to an orthopaedic chap', and we finally went there and we were told it should have been seen years ago.

Marie lived a long way from a main treatment centre, and at that time outreach support workers were very scarce and taken up with caring for people with HIV and AIDS as well as with general family support. She felt she was to blame for not insisting earlier that her son's treatment was not adequate to keep his ankle in good condition, yet she had not had medical training and her medical advisors had not suggested it. Although people in the haemophilia community are expert patients or expert parents, and their expertise is often recognised by their specialists, their limits also need recognition, as does their need for medical support. In new families, that expertise builds slowly, as in Marie's case. There are times when patients, and their parents, do want their doctors to take the lead and exercise their competence as part of a respectful doctor-patient partnership (Jutel 2011, 93).

One way to fill in the gap in support was to call up other parents with children who had similar levels of haemophilia. This, we were told, was often the best way of sharing the responsibility of monitoring and tinkering with the medical treatment required. Many women told us about the support they found as carers through talking to other mothers, such as this mother who told us about it in 1994.

> I had a few parents that I felt comfortable about ringing, just to sound them out to say, 'Would I be making a fool of myself by ringing up the [haemophilia] centre?' And I am also aware that they [haemophilia centre] are really busy and that sometimes I just needed to have a chat.

Support from other parents, from knowledgeable family members, as well as from the Haemophilia Society or Foundation was important in all aspects of caring, from learning how to do injections to dealing with adolescent behaviour. The importance of support to care-giving mothers is a feature widely reported in studies of living with haemophilia, for example an interview study with 13 Swedish carrier mothers of boys with haemophilia (Myrin-Westesson, Baghaei, and Firberg 2013).

One woman drew our attention to the different quality of caring between her earlier role as a care-giving sister to two brothers with haemophilia and her current experience of having a son with haemophilia. Despite these many years of caring for men in her family with haemophilia, she felt emotionally unprepared for caring for her own son:

> Yes, I was informed medically, but perhaps no one can ever express to you...that it is, emotionally and socially ... there are implications as a

parent that you don't face as a sibling … that's not the same as having your own and having to think, 'What's going on?' And having to get up in the middle of the night and try to unfog your brain and look at your son, he's crying, and say, 'Now what's the trouble? …' There's nothing I don't think that can prepare you for the vigilance.

As we described in chapter 2, sensory vigilance expresses clearly what so many mothers told us: constantly listening, observing, feeling for warmth around joints indicating a bleed, and asking carefully devised questions when the child is old enough. One mother told us: 'I can remember that that best sound I ever hear in the morning is to hear [my son] get up and walk evenly. I can tell when he gets up if he's limping, just by his walk'. Some children became adept at covering up their bleeds, at least for a while. Parents had to work to determine if a bleed was going on, without actually asking. Watching a child walking upstairs could show if he was leading with one foot. An older man with haemophilia had devised a good questioning strategy that he told other parents and us about: 'Say, "How long has your knee been sore?"', rather than asking their son if he has a bleed.

Deciding when to treat children with suspected bleeds was part of mothers' caring role, working with their children to get the balance right. This was particularly taxing for mothers with children who had less than severe haemophilia and who therefore were not on prophylaxis. In addition, both parents had to advocate for their child in medical settings especially when they were away from their familiar medical staff. But it was the mothers who tended to write about this in their parent questionnaire or talk about it in interviews.

Adult sons were well aware of the work of caring that their mothers had done. One man who had been brought up on a sheep farm, reminisced about his mother's working life and tried to imagine what it had been like for her. He told a story that had obviously been passed down in his family to illustrate the hard work of care. As well as caring for her two sons with haemophilia, and doing the usual household work, when shearers were on the farm shearing the sheep, his mother also had to prepare morning and afternoon teas for them. These teas were not just a hot drink but included substantial home-baked scones, pikelets, and cakes.

> She'd have me sick, just get me all going again … and [my brother] would get sick and it would be a whole month without any sleep … I remember one day she was getting morning and afternoon tea ready for the men at the woolshed … She must have had 5 or 10 minutes or so and sat down, and of course there was no cup of tea. The old man came steaming over and she'd conked out on the table. She'd gone to sleep. That was our mother.

Siblings, usually sisters, looked out for their brothers, wives for their husbands, and sometimes children kept an eye on their affected parent.

Many of the married and partnered men (two-thirds of the 1994–5 participants over 20 had wives or partners) talked about the difference their wife or partner had made to their lives. Some wives, as key health-keepers (Chambers and Macdonald 1987) in their households, took some responsibility for their husbands' well-being, from suggesting it was time for a treatment through to doing the treatment or caring for the men during periods of ill health or immobility. Several wives were nurses, although few had met their husbands in hospital. Some wives and partners 'helped to fight the battles' for accident compensation or with health authorities. One man wrote: 'my wife is my legs'. He explained that before he was married, he had struggled on with crutches, 'standing on his own two feet', and sustained many bleeds. Sometime after his wedding, he decided to use a wheelchair. After this, his bleeds decreased greatly, and he no longer had to take a lot of time off work. It was his loving relationship with his wife that gave him the confidence to admit that he needed the wheelchair, at least some of the time. This story simultaneously challenges male gender expectations that value independence symbolised by standing on one's own two feet, but also, given that the wheelchair became acceptable only after his marriage, it reinforces these expectations and underlines the crucial importance of the support work of women.

A couple of participants confided that their partners 'did not want to know' about haemophilia. Partners did have to face major challenges, yet the moral and practical support of wives, partners, and other female relatives was mentioned by nearly all adult men as being crucial to their lives and well-being. This was obvious to us at the meetings, camps, conferences and other events that we attended. Many wives showed a watchful but unobtrusive attentiveness. It was laced with a good deal of joking when the time was right, with men admitting to doing somewhat risky things at times, and trying to hide this from their wives.

Women in the haemophilia community had a very wide range of contributions. Their caring, organising, and educating was recognised and celebrated. But many of the women were also people with haemophilia.

Carriers with haemophilia

'I am different, I can't describe it, different to other women'. During an interview in 1995, a woman who experienced bleeding problems struggled to find words to explain her doubts about her own femininity. As the daughter of a man with haemophilia, she had been brought up to believe that only men had haemophilia. Yet she experienced haemophilia-related bleeding problems and therefore, she reasoned, she must be partly male or incompletely female. When Julie turned off the tape recorder, she added that she felt 'like a woman in a man's body'.

Until the mid-1990s, women with haemophilia-related bleeding problems often had difficulty in getting adequate treatment, especially when they had to move outside their known circle of medical specialists because, as Ross (1997, 5) described for Australia, 'no-one believes they have a bleeding problem, especially not one called haemophilia'. Nonspecialist doctors often dismissed women's bleeding problems because of haemophilia's exclusive association with males. For years, women with bleeding due to haemophilia mutations were denied what Nettleton (2006) calls 'permission to be ill'. Haemophilia is rare, many doctors and nurses never have to treat it, and little time is devoted to it in the crowded curricula of medical schools. Only recently has research demonstrated that even carriers who do not notice bleeding problems have joint abnormalities from micro bleeds (CDC 2015). Women most often experienced bleeding difficulties with routine, minor things, like having a boil lanced, whereas more major surgery, which was usually carried out in large hospitals with familiar specialists and blood products available, did not usually present such problems.

Few women mentioned restrictions on playing sport as a problem area for themselves although we asked all women participants if they had bleeding problems and, if so, what effects these had. Even if they knew that they carried the haemophilia mutation, often it was after they had played sport for years that women learned that the bruises or troublesome joints that were such a familiar part of their lives were due to their lowered clotting factor. This was the case for Nola, who had done martial arts, skiing, tennis, and quite a few other sports. As she said, although it was too late for her as a sports-focussed woman in her thirties to undo the damage to her joints, she was empowered by learning at a haemophilia camp that she had mild haemophilia. Until then, she had not made the connection between being a carrier and having all those bruises. In future, she would prevent further damage to herself and, especially, protect her young daughter with mild haemophilia from serious damage by being careful about her choice of physical activities.

Another woman in her late twenties, Sally, was a keen equestrian and participated in several other sports. Sally had made the connection between being a carrier, having mild haemophilia, and all the bruises she got early in life, but it did not deter her despite many accidents, operations, and needing a good deal of physiotherapy. An older woman described how she had played netball in the 1970s, despite having known bleeding problems. Her coach insisted on all the goal posts being padded, and she played on regardless of bruises. She laughed that 'Everyone else thought we were a wussy team'. Rugby also figured in a young participant's life, but she recalled only one bad knock when a much heavier girl fell on top of her during a tackle, resulting in a headache (sounding like concussion). Although rugby was 'pretty good' (an understatement of how much she enjoyed it) she accepted that she could not play it competitively and be safe. Tennis and several other sports were mentioned by women, but when they talked about their bleeding problems they were much more likely to talk about menstruation, nose-bleeds, dental work, and childbirth as the main problems, not sport.

Despite its popularity, women's sport did not carry the same emotional freight for women with low factor levels that it did for men. This can be explained by the cultural salience of men's (not women's) sport, the emphasis on women as carriers rather than people with haemophilia, and the relatively mild levels of haemophilia for most women, which allow considerable leeway in physical activities.

Only a tiny minority of women had severe problems with bleeding, but this rarity caused them even greater difficulty. Gillian, the mother of a young girl whose expression of the haemophilia mutation indicated severe haemophilia, initially had a difficult time, both in getting information and in obtaining services for her daughter's bleeding. When we first met her in 1995, her daughter was still young.

> There are so few women and girls recognised as having haemophilia that everything is very male orientated ... I find it a bit frustrating.... My daughter doesn't realise that she's the only girl [with severe haemophilia], and it's going to be hard for her when she does realise that.

The efforts of women to have their or their daughter's bleeding issues recognised, named, and treated as haemophilia indicated the importance of diagnostic consonance in doctor-patient relationships (Jutel 2011, 62). However, in this case, the struggle was not to recognise a new disorder but to overcome the genetic deterministic idea that because haemophilia was X-chromosome linked, that only men, whose Y chromosome could not protect them from the expression of the gene mutation, could have it. The stories of genetic sex and cultural gender of men as active bleeders fitted so closely that there was little room for the recognition that women could bleed too. It took changes in scientific understandings of genetic expression and in gendered habitus (Bourdieu 2002), as well as specific action by the women concerned, for women's bleeding to be acknowledged.

In the first phases of our research, most women with bleeding problems whom we met felt they were invisible in the haemophilia community. Nearly all of them felt isolated and many unknowingly had in common that their embodied knowledge of haemophilia was disputed by health care providers. Because these women were so few and scattered around the country, they did not have the comfort of knowing that other women shared these experiences. This became very apparent during our interviews. One young woman in her late teens said, 'I really don't know how to describe the isolation. If you had other women to talk to and could say, "What's it like for you, and how do you feel when this happens? [that would help]"'. When we offered to put this person in touch with the woman who felt 'like a woman in a man's body,' we found that both leapt at the opportunity for mutual support and discussion.

Because the existing discourse excluded women as bleeders, not only did some women have doubts about their own femininity, but the younger women were unsure about what it really meant for them, especially regarding having children. A woman in her thirties who had a partner, but had decided not to have children, explained her decision during an interview in 1995:

> I didn't want to go through what I imagined would be fearful child-birth. So, I decided way back that a family wasn't for me ... [but] perhaps way back, had I the right contacts and reassurance, my life may have gone in a different direction.

As late as the 1980s, women had been offered hysterectomies when they were in their teens or early twenties as a way of coping with being 'expressed carriers' and having excessive menstrual bleeding. A mother told us in 1995, 'Doctors wanted to give her a hysterectomy when she was 15 and she told them she was not even sexually active yet and it was too big a decision to make at her age'. A few women eventually did have hysterectomies, often after one or two children, because the almost constant (up to three weeks long) heavy periods led to anaemia and other problems.

Over the latter part of the 1990s and into the twenty-first century, the value of contact between women with bleeding problems, the seriousness of bleeding problems for women, the possibilities for specific treatment for women's distressing menstrual bleeding, and preventative attention during birthing, gained much more attention (e.g., Huszti and Cooksey 1996; Paper 1993; Ross 1997; Park 2005). This was true in the international haemophilia community, as reflected in the programmes at successive World Congresses and in New Zealand, where the photos from successive years on the HFNZ website (www.haemophilia.org.nz) tell this story of recognition. At national haemophilia camps, including camps specifically for women, and in the HFNZ Newsletter, *Bloodline,* women's issues were on the programme. Women expressed great satisfaction at what they learned from sharing their knowledge and experience with others. Through these sessions, many women realised that they too had bleeding problems. By the end of the decade they had learned that their bleeding could be treated through a variety of options. In 1999, during a family interview, a woman reflected:

> Knowledge is empowering, isn't it? And just the sharing. There was one woman there [at the camp a year before] and we talked about it afterwards, this woman and I, and she said that when she has her periods—I didn't realise the other woman had it too—she'd actually have to call out for her husband to pass her a towel ... And you realise that there are other women out there who have that predicament.

The general silence about menstruation among generations of New Zealand women (Smith 1991, 91) probably contributed to the silencing of women with haemophilia in their monthly struggles with prolonged and heavy bleeding. One woman told Kathryn at a haemophilia camp in 1998 that, although she talked to her best friend about 'everything', she 'wouldn't have a clue' what her periods were like, how long or heavy. There was little chance of comparison with such a cloak of silence. Women had accepted as normal the bleeding and bruising that was a result of having reduced clotting factor levels: just something they had to put up with. This is a further example of the discourse of stoicism: 'you just get on with it' (Beasley 2003, 172), expected of and espoused by New Zealand women. The silence was deepened by the focus of attention on men's pressing needs, especially in relation to the trauma of the blood-borne infections. Besides these life and death struggles, heavy periods might appear trivial: hardly worth a mention, even though they caused pain, anaemia, and were socially disabling. These values influenced the local biology of women's experience of haemophilia.

A woman who had read our initial report (Park *et al.* 1995) told us after a meeting in 2003 how much she had enjoyed reading about 'carrier women', as 'that issue had been swept under the carpet'. She reflected that while growing up, she had always been 'the sister' to her brothers with their bleeding crises and now she was 'the mother' of a boy with haemophilia. Despite low clotting factor levels, she was not recognised as a person/patient in her own right, no one paid her any attention, nor did she think of herself as someone that might need looking after. In hindsight she was horrified about what might have happened to her or her babies during her home births: haemorrhages and intracranial bleeds.

Despite the increasing recognition that women, too, may have bleeding problems, this recognition is by no means universal. Even in the two update studies in 1999 and 2006, we found women who were just discovering, or had struggles convincing others, that women could also have coagulation difficulties. But these struggles were now largely outside the haemophilia community. In an emergency department in 1999, Elizabeth was asked about family history when she took in her daughter with suspected concussion; she reported they had haemophilia in the family and she did not know her daughter's clotting factor levels.

ELIZABETH: Yes, my son's a haemophiliac.
DOCTOR: She's a girl. It only happens with boys, you know.
ELIZABETH: Yes, I know, I've got a haemophilia boy.
DOCTOR: Well what are you worried about?
ELIZABETH: Because she has undiagnosed possible carrier status and carriers also have lowered levels of factor eight (FVIII).
DOCTOR: Oh no, but it only happens to boys.

Elizabeth was confident in her own knowledge, but she and her daughter were 'dismissed' by the doctor who *knew* that 'it only happens to boys'. Fortunately for women, such stories are by no means as frequent as they used to be. Nola, in 2006, had recently come to realise that both she and her daughter were 'symptomatic carriers', which, as noted above, explained her own arthritic joints.

NOLA: My daughter has a clotting factor level of 20 per cent.

J: Oh, OK, she's got more or less mild haemophilia, then.

NOLA: Yes, she basically has. That's what they consider 'symptomatic carrier'. Basically, she is a haemophiliac but because it is not so well known in females, then they call her that.

J: Yeah, what do you think about that?

NOLA: I think it sucks! And she does too. Just because it's kind of, understanding, people don't think that females can be haemophiliacs. We didn't know until my daughter was diagnosed. ... That kind of makes things a lot more difficult because we don't have the support that we need, and even people within the Haemophilia Foundation themselves don't really recognise us, so I found that a lot of the [Young Families] Camp was great, but I didn't find out a lot of the stuff that was more important to us.

The young women's workshops were designed specifically for people like Nola, but the changes they signal are slow and incremental for the haemophilia community and for the health system. In 2005, Frances who had factor IX haemophilia, had what she described as 'a little battle', with PHARMAC. She had experienced severe menstrual problems for some years that caused other health issues, and was concerned with being on the birth control pill for long periods of time. She was ably assisted by the HFNZ outreach worker in a successful negotiation to have haemophilia listed as one of the conditions under which the Mirena® IUD device, which supplies small quantities of hormone directly in the uterus, could be supplied free to the patient. Five years before, she had had to pay for it herself.

This is the kind of incremental change, that, looking back over a 15-year span, Gillian, the mother of a daughter with haemophilia, saw as 'huge'. But it does not happen by itself. As Gillian said, some of the difference is 'because I've banged on about it so much!', her way of saying she has challenged the accepted narratives. Small acts like using inclusive gender pronouns, using 'haemophilia' for both men and women with reduced clotting factor levels, efforts to educate nonspecialists, and attention to lobbying for services and systems were all necessary, as well as the medical research and the education based on it, to better understand the reasons and mechanisms for women's bleeding problems.

Women 'carriers' are no longer as silent or silenced about their own bleeding problems when they occur. As a result, more individual women with bleeding problems are being identified and more recognition is being accorded to women's bleeding. Thus, to those more traditional areas for which women have long been valued, i.e., caring at home for and about family members with bleeding problems, and taking responsibility for family planning, a new dimension has been added: women as people who may bleed from haemophilia.

Conclusion: gendered changes and different haemophilias

An elderly gentleman and long-term member of the haemophilia community said in 1999:

> I hadn't thought about it before, but both men and women did carry haemophilia and maybe we should be thinking about both men and women with haemophilia, although it affects them both in different ways.

Later that year in an interview, Susan who was a mother of children with and without haemophilia said,

> it's not just the boys that are bleeders, they are also carriers … For years … it has been known that the man with haemophilia will carry it to his daughter, and yet that's not discussed. And the automatic blame that the woman has to carry.

It still comes as a surprise to some men—now, mainly the partners of women carriers who often find learning about haemophilia a challenge—to learn that their boys with haemophilia will pass it on to their daughters. We have been at numerous meetings over the years, including one in January 2006 at which the following exchange took place, where that particular penny has dropped. It happened at an informal educational session. A father of a little boy with haemophilia asked a question after listening to a haemophilia specialist talk about various options for having children: 'You mean that if my son has daughters, they might have haemophilia?' He was met with a chorus from the audience, confirmed by the speaker, 'No, they *will* have haemophilia!' The father looked very taken aback. As Susan, cited at the beginning of this section, noted, the everyday stories of haemophilia tend to mask this fact of men being carriers. Even when men clearly realised they also could pass haemophilia on and took preventative steps, the matter was seldom discussed. However, there were a few exceptions.

One of these was an older man with mild haemophilia, James, who had never married or had children, who described in 1994 how when he was a young man, his doctor told him 'never to marry and have kids'. A few other men had been similarly advised, but most had ignored it. James had never discussed this with his natal family, but he told the following story:

> It became a fixation and I carried this idea right through farming. I started breeding pedigree sheep … The first year I was running round flat out lambing some of these ewes. Well, that [i.e., ewes having problems with lambing and therefore needing the farmer's help] is very often hereditary, so the next year I said I'm not going to do this. Any ewe that has lambing problems I will shoot. So that is what I did and I shot half the ewes. The neighbours thought I was crazy, but from then on, I had no problems [with lambing].

As a person with mild haemophilia, who was a flower breeder in his retirement, James's decision not to have children was made for similar reasons to good stock or flower breeding: to ensure there were 'no problems' for future generations. Sadly, he added that if he had known then what he knew as an older person about haemophilia and its treatment, he would have decided differently about having a family as a young man.

The genetics of haemophilia mean that men will not have boys with haemophilia. They will transmit it to all daughters, most of whom will not have serious bleeding problems. This delay of a generation in the usual expression of haemophilia makes men's role in its transmission less of a point of discussion and often completely masks it. Cultural understandings of reproduction, which despite what we all 'know', still allow us to say colloquially in New Zealand, 'she got herself pregnant', also play an important part in assigning reproduction to women only. But also significant is the emphasis on men as actors which, in the haemophilia community, translates into an overwhelming focus on men as bleeders to the exclusion, until very recent years, of their role in passing on haemophilia.

Within the haemophilia community what Rich (1980) called 'compulsory heterosexuality' has been dominant. We have never made this theme the focus of direct enquiry. Assumed heterosexuality is embedded in many aspects of life in that community, whether it be rugby conversations, discussions among young men about when and how to tell a girlfriend that you have haemophilia or hepatitis C, or among parents about the best time to tell their daughters that they are or might be carriers, and all the discussions among carriers about having children. Despite this, there appears to be complete recognition and acceptance of gay community members and their partners, including electing them as foundation officers. Such openness is part of broader societal trends exemplified by the recognition of same-sex marriage equality.

In the early years, we speculated that because HIV was connected with men having sex with men, and men with haemophilia had contracted HIV through clotting factor replacement products, an emphasis on the heterosexuality of men with haemophilia was a way of maintaining a separate identity within the shared tragedy of HIV and AIDS and then hepatitis C. Such a factor is likely to be a minor contributor, however. More likely, culturally dominant male gender roles, rather than heterosexuality per se, are most relevant. The goal of 'living a normal life', so often expressed by men with haemophilia, included for them being able to work, to play sport, to establish a long-term partnership or marriage, to be able to contribute to the support of one's family and to have children and hopefully, grandchildren. It seems significant that a man who was content to get around in a wheelchair was able to relinquish standing on his own two feet only after he had married a loving, supportive woman.

As discussed, many women in the haemophilia community have their own bleeding problems. These have specific repercussions for women that are often quite different from those experienced by men. In addition to bruising and bleeding like men with mild haemophilia, women have particular issues over menstruation or childbirth, difficulties relating to securing adequate treatment and even for gender identity. These repercussions are always experienced in particular gendered contexts. As we have observed, women's practices of silence, stoicism, and always putting the men first has been changing.

Some of the change in women's haemophilia over the last two decades can be attributed to broader societal gender change. With the flow-on effects of the women's movement, silences were broken around many aspects of women's lives and women learned to question always putting themselves last. Commercial interests of companies providing 'feminine products' and medications, the pervasiveness of advertising of such products on TV and in magazines, and the more general medicalisation of aspects of women's lives, from menstruation to menopause and beyond, interacted with these changing values. Language to discuss aspects of the workings of women's bodies became more readily available in the general community, and in the haemophilia context, women felt empowered to question their experiences and to seek assistance.

At the same time, and as a result of the women's movement, and the availability of better contraception and legal abortion, women had greater control over whether and when they became mothers. The allocation of domestic work also changed somewhat. Husbands and partners were expected to share more in the responsibilities of parenting and the roles of men beyond just breadwinners became more emphasised while their female partners' breadwinning contributions became more necessary. These trends were not universal but pervade discourses and sometimes, but not as often as many women would like, practices, of parenting and household chores. People in the haemophilia community were part of it. Although women were still centrally involved in the enactment of haemophilia as caregivers and carriers, some space was created for them to be people with their own bleeding problems. This change parallels complementary changes in men's enactment of haemophilia.

We suggest that some of the explanation of these changes is specific to the haemophilia community. The epidemics of HIV and hepatitis C within this community to a large extent put other issues into abeyance from the 1980s on, as community members attended to the pressing issues of the day. In the latter part of the 1990s, some energy and space was created for other things to be addressed, including women's issues, and indeed issues of biculturalism as we discuss in our concluding chapters. Newly appointed outreach workers and our own 1994–5 study found that there were a number of women with haemophilia scattered around the country, many isolated and confused. One or two of these were advocates on their own and their children's behalf, and kept the profile of women's bleeding and carrier issues in the forefront. In the New Zealand and international haemophilia communities, women started speaking out. For example, a number of specific workshops or sessions were convened: the Pacific Rim workshop on Carrier Perspectives in 1997 (Ross 1997), an Irish Workshop on Women's Bleeding Issues in 2003, and designated sessions on women's bleeding at successive World Congresses (e.g., 2006). The website of the Canadian Hemophilia Society (2018) forthrightly states that some women have mild haemophilia, although it is rare, the Hemophilia Federation of America has a webpage 'Women Bleed Too! Toolkit' (2018) and in 2012 WFH published *Carriers and Women with Hemophilia*, a brief informational booklet that distinguishes between all women who carry haemophilia, and those who both carry and have low clotting factor levels, i.e., haemophilia. Medical, psychological, and social research on haemophilia has also added to understandings of women's issues in the haemophilia community. Through these internal community changes, in conjunction with more general social change, women's own needs and issues had more opportunity to be articulated and addressed, creating different haemophilias for women over time.

Returning to the rugby idiom, women's active role in haemophilia has come in from the sidelines, just as women's rugby also now shares some of the limelight alongside men's. Simultaneously, as masculinity has become less restrictive in the wider society, men's roles in reproducing haemophilia and in supporting their partners in their decisions have also become more visible and accepted. The active-male-rugby-player versus the passive-female-sacrificial-caregiver gendered enactments of haemophilia were more evident when we first began our research, but these have been modified, becoming more complex and less binary as time has gone on. These social changes occurred alongside rapid changes in the technologies relating to haemophilia. Changes in treatment technologies were important in relation to the ability to achieve 'normal' life and gendered expectations, but perhaps even more important were the changing technologies relating to reproduction, to having families. It is to these we turn in the next chapter, as we add further complexity to the story of different haemophilias and the complex interactions between biology, science, and other social and cultural frameworks.

Notes

1. The Whitehall studies researched health inequalities among British Civil Servants, see for example, Marmot *et al.* (1991).
2. The chances of women having two affected X chromosomes are remote, due to haemophilia's rarity.
3. A possible explanation for this is that doctors reassured men with haemophilia that their children would not have it (i.e., their boys would not have haemophilia, or carry the gene for it). The men may have overlooked the fact that all their daughters would carry the gene.

References

Beasley, A. 2003. '"You Just Get on with It": Taboo, Stoicism and the Body Politic— The Menopause Experience among Three Cohorts of New Zealand Women'. *SITES (NS)* 1 (1):160–85.

Belich, J., and L. Wevers. 2008. 'Understanding New Zealand Cultural Identities'. Discussion paper prepared by the Stout Research Centre for New Zealand Studies for the Ministry of Culture and Heritage. Wellington: Victoria University.

Benseman, J., and J. Park. 1998. 'Bleeding Nuisance: The Implications of Haemophilia for Education'. *Australasian Journal of Special Education* 21 (2):81–97.

Bourdieu, P. 2002. *Masculine Domination*. Translated by R. Nice. Stanford: Stanford University Press.

Butler, J. 1990. *Gender Trouble: Feminism and the Subversion of Identity*. New York: Routledge.

Canadian Hemophilia Society. 2018. 'What is Hemophilia? Who is Affected by hemophilia?' https://www.hemophilia.ca/what-is-hemophilia#ca10ba60b6818d2f7 (last accessed 11 Nov, 2018).

CDC. 2015. 'New Study Findings: Research Study Shows that Female Hemophilia Carriers Have Evidence of Joint Abnormalities'. http://www.fwgbd.org/news/new-study-findings-research-shows-female-hemophilia-carriers-have-evidence-of-joint-abnormalities (last accessed 11 Nov, 2018).

Chambers, A., and J. Macdonald. 1987. *For Health's Sake: Women's Health-Keeping in Central Auckland*. Department of Anthropology, University of Auckland.

Connell, R.W. 1987. *Gender and Power: Society, the Person and Sexual Politics*. Stanford: Stanford University Press.

De Jong, P. 1987. '"The Old Rugby Grows on You": The Making of a Game in a Small New Zealand Town'. *SITES* 14:35–56.

Desmarais, F. 2004. 'Sport as a Moralizing Device in New Zealand Television Advertising Discourse'. Dept. of Management Communication Working Paper Series, University of Waikato.

Douglas, M. 1970. *Natural Symbols: Explorations in Cosmology*. Barrie & Rockliff: Cresset Press.

Fougere, G. 1989. 'Sport, Culture, and Identity: The Case of Rugby Football'. In *Culture and Identity in New Zealand*, edited by D. Novitz, and B. Willmott, 110–12. Wellington: GP Books.

Hochschild, A.R. 1979. 'Emotion Work, Feeling Roles, and Social Structure'. *American Journal of Sociology* 85:551–75.

Husxti, H.C., and D. Cooksey. 1996. 'Weekend Retreat for Teenage Women with Bleeding Disorders'. Paper presented at the World Federation of Haemophilia Conference Presentation, Dublin, June 23–8.

Joll, K. 2005. 'Physiotherapy and Exercise in Haemophilia'. Hamilton: Waikato Hospital.

Jones, M. 2008. 'Measuring Passive Childcare in Time Use Surveys: A Comparison of International Methodologies'. www.stats.govt.nz.

Jutel, A.G. 2011. *Putting a Name to it: Diagnosis in Contemporary Society*. Baltimore: Johns Hopkins University Press.

Kaufert, P.A. 1999. 'The Vanishing Woman: Gender and Population Health'. *In Sex, Gender and Health*, edited by T.M. Pollard, and S.B. Hyatt, 118–36. Cambridge: Cambridge University Press.

Lewis, N., and G. Winder. 2007. 'Sporting Narratives and Globalisation: Making Links between the All Black Tours of 1905 and 2005'. *New Zealand Geographer* 63 (3):202–15.

Lupton, D. 1994. *Medicine as Culture: Illness, Disease and the Body in Western Societies*. London: Sage.

McCaw, R., with McGee, G. 2012. *The Open Side*. Auckland: Hachette Livre NZ Ltd.

MacDonald, R. 1996. *The Game of Our Lives: The Story of Rugby and New Zealand—and How They've Shaped Each Other*. Auckland: Viking.

Marmot, M.G., G.D. Davey-Smith, S. Stansfield, C. Patel, F. North, J. Head, I. White, E. Brunner, and A. Feeney. 1991. 'Health Inequalities Among British Civil Servants: The Whitehall II Study'. *Lancet* 337 (8754):1387–93.

Mol, A. 2002. *The Body Multiple: Ontology in Medical Practice*. Durham: Duke University Press.

Myrin-Westesson, L., F. Baghaei, and F. Friberg. 2013. 'The Experience of Being a Female Carrier of Haemophilia and the Mother of a Haemophilic Child'. *Haemophilia* 19:219–24.

Nettleton, S. 2006. '"I Just Want Permission to be Ill": Towards a Sociology of Medically Unexplained Symptoms'. *Social Science & Medicine* 62:1167–78.

New Zealand Herald 31 July–4 August 2008. Items Concerning Rugby. A1.

Ortner, S. 1973. 'On Key Symbols'. *American Anthropologist* 75 (5):1338–46.

Palenski, R. 2015. *Rugby: A New Zealand History*. Auckland: Auckland University Press.

Paper, R. 1993. 'Females Bleed Too!'. *HANDI Quarterly* 3:1–9.

Park, J. 2000. '"The Only Hassle is You Can't Play Rugby": Haemophilia and Masculinity in New Zealand'. *Current Anthropology* 41:443–52.

Park, J. 2005. 'Beyond "His Sisters and His Cousins and His Aunts": Discourses of Haemophilia and Women's Experiences in New Zealand'. In *A Polymath Anthropologist: Essays in Honour of Ann Chowning*, RAL 6, edited by C. Gross, H.D. Lyons, and D.A. Counts, 97–104. Auckland: University of Auckland.

Park, J., K. Scott, J. Benseman, and E. Berry. 1995. *A Bleeding Nuisance: Living with Haemophilia in Aotearoa New Zealand*. Department of Anthropology, University of Auckland.

Phillips, J. 1987. *A Man's Country? The Image of the Pakeha Male, a History*. Auckland: Penguin Books.

Pringle, R. 2002. 'Living the Contradictions: A Foucauldian Examination of my Youthful Rugby Experiences'. In *The Life of Brian: Masculinities, Sexualities and Health in New Zealand*, edited by H. Worth, A. Paris, and L. Allen, 57–72. Dunedin: University of Otago Press.

Rich, A. 1980. 'Compulsory Heterosexuality and Lesbian Existence'. *Signs: Journal of Women in Culture and Society* 5 (4):631–60.

Ross, J. 1997. 'The Perspectives of Haemophilia Carriers'. World Federation of Hemophilia Pacific Rim Workshop Papers 8:1–7.

Ryan, G. ed. 2005. *Tackling Rugby Myths: Rugby and New Zealand Society 1854-2004*. Dunedin: University of Otago Press.

Smith, R. 1991. 'Who am I? Identity'. In *Ladies a Plate: Change and Continuity in the Lives of New Zealand Women*, edited by J. Park, 60–95. Auckland: Auckland University Press.

Statistics New Zealand. 1996. *1996 Census of Population and Dwellings*. Wellington: Statistics New Zealand.

Women Bleed Too! Toolkit. 2018. http://www.hemophiliafed.org/for-patient-families/resources/toolkits/women-bleed-too-toolkit/ (last accessed 11 Nov, 2018).

[WFH] World Federation of Hemophilia. 2012. 'Carriers and Women with Hemophilia'. http://www.wfh.org (last accessed 11 Nov, 2018).

4 New networks and technologies of care
Different haemophilias

The difference that time makes

> I was about 14, 15. For about four months they kept you in traction [in hospital]. The bleed had ceased.... It was just crazy. Then they had this idea of putting my leg in a calliper, and of course that was the worst thing they could have done because the muscle just wasted away.... One time I went away on holiday [to my uncle's farm] and we all went for a swim in the river... so I ripped [the calliper] off and chucked it into the bushes. It is probably still there, rusting away.
>
> (Colin, an older man in 1995, describing the care offered in his boyhood in the 1950s.)

With no clotting factor and few diagnostic tools, a range of networks and technologies of care were used to try to stop Colin's bleeding and prevent new bleeds from starting. These included hospital care from which parents were almost excluded, rest, traction, hydrotherapy, heat to reduce bleed masses, physiotherapy, and callipers. The networks of care brought into play here included the hospital staff mentioned as 'they' but also manufacturers of traction equipment, splint makers, and boot makers.

Care is a concept with an ever-broadening range of meanings 'involving care for, care of and care about' (Park and Fitzgerald 2011, 426). While care may frequently entail positive affect and gentle treatment, it also contains the seeds of worry and may suggest loss of autonomy, as in 'being taken into care'. Mol (2008) suggests that the language of care in Western medicine has been silenced, permitting rational choice and efficiency discourses to dominate. Networks and technologies of care are complex and need analysis in their own contexts to fully comprehend how biopower is exercised in each case. In this chapter, we explore how an ethics of care is intertwined with liberal discourses of choice and with marketisation.

Colin shared with us an extract from his hospital notes, a letter of 30 May 1950 from his provincial hospital specialist to the specialist in the metropolitan hospital: 'I feel it unlikely that any effective treatment is possible but, in view of his age [5 years], one feels that all possible should be done'.

As this letter shows, the networks of care extended well beyond the local. This letter was sent decades before the construct of 'quality adjusted life years' (Weinstein, Torrance, and McGuire 2009) was invented and it is difficult to interpret now, but it seems likely that it expresses both caring and compassion for a five-year-old living a painful life.

We discuss two types of networks and technologies of care: first those involved in the treatment of haemophilia and then those involved in testing for haemophilia. Like the dimensions discussed in chapters 2 and 3, changing biotechnologies and networks of care interconnect with haemophilia as a biosocial condition to produce further different haemophilias. We use 'networks of care' to refer to the overarching links and nodes consisting of seen and unseen human and nonhuman entities, such as companies or spiritual beings. 'Technologies of care' refers to networks of knowledge, conventional practices, material objects, and the meanings with which they are imbued, which together create apparently coherent entities used in networks of care (Brodwin 2000; Latour 1987). Networks and technologies of care are mutually constitutive. We ask how materiality and meaning interact at nodal points in these networks, and with what consequences for daily lives of people living with haemophilia.

What studies of living with haemophilia or other conditions can do is to show how changing technologies are part of what makes up haemophilia for people with it and for those around them. Whether people with haemophilia envisage themselves as 'bold guinea pigs' for scientific experiments (discussed later) or 'moral pioneers' making moral decisions that have not had to be made before (Rapp 1991, 1993), or in quite other terms, they deal on a daily basis with the legacies of scientific breakthroughs in the areas of reproduction, treatment, testing for haemophilia status and the ever-promising gene therapy. It is these changing networks and technologies and haemophilias that are explored in this chapter.

Each of the nodes in Colin's care network had its own networks, as Latour (1987) has described. For example, the hospital staff were organised in a uniformed medical and nursing hierarchy, and supported by clerical and housekeeping staff, orderlies, and so on. These staff used various items of equipment and these too were connected to factories, labs, and raw materials in an almost infinite regression. Equipment, the stethoscope perhaps being the most famous, was meaningful, declaring some staff clinical and others ancillary. All these networks were brought into being and into association, becoming the technologies used at the time, and in turn creating the haemophilia of the moment, as Mol (2002) and many others have argued. In Colin's story, it was the kind of haemophilia where you had to stay in traction for months, a lonely kid in hospital, and afterward had to wear a calliper, and put up with terrible pain and problems with getting about. With this kind of haemophilia, parents were relegated to being visitors while their son was in hospital. But at home, they were the primary caregivers. Colin himself was an active agent in his care, jettisoning the callipers to become more physically active.

Fast forward approximately 50 years. A mother, in 1995, described the then-current approach to the care of her young son, David, at the Auckland haemophilia centre. The family had travelled there from their hometown to get more specialist advice and treatment after receiving the best care their local hospital could provide.

> We get to Auckland and [the paediatric haematologist] has [the joint bleed] under control within a couple of days. I mean everything was perfect. We had splints, we had ideas, we had exercises to do, anything to better it—swimming, using the muscles to try and [support the joints]—and that's what we wanted to do.

Here, parents are active agents in the network of care at home and in hospital, bringing their son to Auckland in their effort to do the best for their child. Like Colin's physician, they were extending the network of care. In Auckland, they meet a very rare (for New Zealand) specialist, a paediatric haematologist, part of a multidisciplinary team involved in haemophilia care and, like his colleagues, a product of years of training and experience, with a passion for haemophilia. Other members of the team are the haemophilia nurse and the physiotherapist and eventually, when David is ready to go home, the NZHS outreach worker. The parents too are part of the team: 'we had ideas, we had exercises to do'. David is cared for as an outpatient, accompanied by his parents, and is given sufficient clotting factor replacement to stem the bleeding, which had not been managed effectively. David does not need to put up with bleeding and pain. He himself, through exercise, and later through learning to administer his own treatment products, is also part of the team in his lifelong care.

David's treatment product connects with a whole network of blood banks, blood donors, blood processors, and all the background research and management that goes into that. The hospital is, in 1995, a complex organisation, part of a regionalised health system, funded by a central Ministry of Health. Complex behind-the-scenes accounting transactions are necessary for David to get this care in Auckland. This is a different haemophilia from Colin's. But some things have not changed. Swimming, as Colin discovered for himself, is a great sport for kids with haemophilia. At times joints have to be supported: but in 1995, they were supported temporarily with light composite splints. And boys quite often continue to not do what they are told, sometimes with good effects, as in Colin doffing his callipers, sometimes not.

Technologies and the devices that are part of them are products of particular historical processes and derive some meaning from their history as well as from the social, cultural, gendered, and biological contexts with which they are in productive interaction. Callipers, for example, invoke polio for Julie as her father contracted it in the 1916 epidemic. Splints or the use of ice might evoke household or sporting accidents. The development of all these technologies creates new dilemmas for people with haemophilia, changing—in sometimes subtle, sometimes dramatic, ways—the experience of haemophilia for people with it, their families and their health workers. As an example, June describes the new haemophilia created by home treatment—a haemophilia that meant her son could participate much more.

KATHRYN: What's the difference between treating at home and not treating at home?

JUNE: Not treating at home? Yesterday morning [son] had a bleed before he went to school. I started treatment at a quarter to nine, by 9 o'clock we were finished. We were a quarter of an hour late for school. Before, in the past, when [son] had a bleed, I could look at five or six hours at the hospital. (Mother in 1995)

Treatment and testing technologies and their networks of care may be theorised as forms of biopower. The concept of biopower advanced by Rabinow and Rose is a more precise one than that of some other theorists. It has three crucial elements:

> ... truth discourses about the 'vital' character of living human beings and an array of authorities considered competent to speak that truth; ... Strategies for intervention upon collective existence in the name of life and health ... Modes of subjectification, through which individuals are brought to work on themselves ... in the name of their own [or others'] life and health.
>
> (Rabinow and Rose 2006, 197)

Treatment technologies help produce people with haemophilia as contributing members of society, and/or as brave, risk-taking pioneers, especially in relation to trials of gene therapy, or perhaps, as a population more or less deserving of help from the public purse, and of attention from pharmaceutical companies. The embryo or foetal selection that some technologies involve may invoke a painful history of eugenics, vitriolic abortion debates, and fears of science gone mad, while at the same time they derive meaning from their current contributions to the hope of producing healthy babies, reducing misery and grief, and opening new markets for pharmaceutical companies.

One major change in the networks of care between the generations of Colin and David is in the quality of the relationships of care. Where formerly, especially outside the circle of haematologists, many patients and parents were at the lower stratum of a hierarchy and expected to do what they were told by clinical caregivers, by 1995, parents and patients were recognised as expert partners in care, in a relationship that extended well beyond the hospital.

Technologies for treatment

Haemophilia clotting factor replacement products derived from human blood were initially received as a great gift (Titmuss 1970). A middle-aged man in 1995 declared: 'The supply of factor VIII changed my life. Up to 1968, any bleed was treated with bed rest and bandages'. He went on to say that clotting factor replacement therapy had enabled him to get an education, enjoy his job, and live a normal life. Even though blood products had given him HIV and hepatitis C, he was still convinced that the advantages of factor VIII outweighed the disadvantages. This starkly highlights the poor quality of his life before 1968.

After viral contamination, many people with haemophilia regarded factor VIII and IX products as dangerous or potentially dangerous, well beyond the time after which they were technically safe. In 1995, at least two years after hepatitis C had been excluded from the blood supply, a mother described experiencing 'an invisible hurdle' when starting on a new batch of treatment products from a new set of donors. She would think to herself, 'Oh God, here we go, a new batch of blood products, what's in this lot, is it OK?'.

Part of this network of care was the relationship of people with haemophilia to the state: they had lost trust in a 'government [which] has stuffed up twice', as a man with hepatitis C told us in 1995. Even in 2006, when the blood supply had been known to be safe for well over a decade, several people confessed to having a residual worry about product safety. Nita, the mother of the boy with complex haemophilia and delayed diagnosis who was introduced in chapter 2, was one. Her son used blood-derived products because of his treatment complications and Nita had that '0.01 per cent' of residual fear. Viral contamination and fear of this contamination gave rise to new haemophilias and created acceptance or enthusiasm for the new recombinant clotting products and later, other genetic therapies.

For men and women with a haemophilia mutation who know that they can pass it on to the next generation, 'carrying haemophilia' is also different from the past because of these new treatment and care networks and technologies. Most members of the younger generations said that haemophilia was no longer 'serious enough' to warrant the avoidance of passing it on, despite the availability of a range of tests and procedures to assist giving birth to babies without haemophilia. Thus, different haemophilias also affected people's subsequent embrace of new technologies. The mutually constructed haemophilia-technology relationship is on-going.

One woman, Lynette, with boys with haemophilia, discussed various technologies with Julie one day as they sat in the sun in a rest period during a haemophilia camp. We chuckled as she proclaimed that people with haemophilia are 'guinea pigs who boldly go where no pig has gone before'. This invocation of the brave heroes of Star Trek coupled with the image of passivity evoked by the lab guinea pig neatly subverted the erasure of people with haemophilia in medical breakthrough narratives, but at the same time it posed their dilemmas. People with haemophilia are reliant on and mostly hopeful for technological innovations, but they are the ones who have to decide to use them or not, and they bear the consequences. They surely partake in an economy of hope and fear.

A history: from snake venom and peanuts to clotting factor concentrates

Haemophilia treatment and scientific understanding of that remarkable tissue, human blood, have gone hand in hand. Bleeding disorders were recognised in the ancient world and recorded in both Jewish and Arabic medical writings. The first detailed modern descriptions were penned in the 1790s and 1800s, but the term 'haemophilia' was first used in a medical treatise in 1828. In 1938, the deficiency in what is now called factor VIII (FVIII) was discovered, but it was not until 1952 that factor IX (FIX) was discovered (National Hemophilia Foundation [NHF] 2018a). Various remedies were tried, including snake venom, which enhanced clotting and was referred to by several of our older participants as a treatment they were aware of. Large amounts of peanut products also had a positive effect on clotting. Home remedies featured. For example, an older man described how he had suffered from bleeds to the throat when he was young. Under medical supervision, his home treatment was an iced leather collar around his neck and hot water bottles to his feet 'to draw the blood away'. For other bleeds, most often in legs and arms, bed rest with elevation of the affected area if possible, splints to try and protect vulnerable joints, ice, bandaging, and pain relief were all part of the treatment process.

With advances in knowledge of blood transfusion, blood groups and the potential for the development of antibodies, the stage was set for advances in haemophilia treatment in the first part of the twentieth century. At first, treatment was with whole blood, later with plasma (1936) which was fractionated at specific temperatures (from 1944) to produce the different factors essential to clotting. The coagulation cascade, which refers to the complex interactions of different proteins acting in sequence that promote the formation of a clot, was first described in 1964 (see Figures 4.1 and 4.2) (Canadian Hemophilia Society 2018; NHF 2018a).

In 1965, the concentration of FVIII as a result of slow thawing of frozen plasma (cryoprecipitate) was discovered and within a decade, concentrates became widely available, although cryoprecipitate was eventually superseded by a range of other antihaemophilic products, freeze-dried from pooled plasma. These developments afforded the possibility of home treatment from the mid-1970s (WFH 2015). Clotting factors work as part of the coagulation cascade in complex interactions, as the World Federation of Hemophilia website explains.

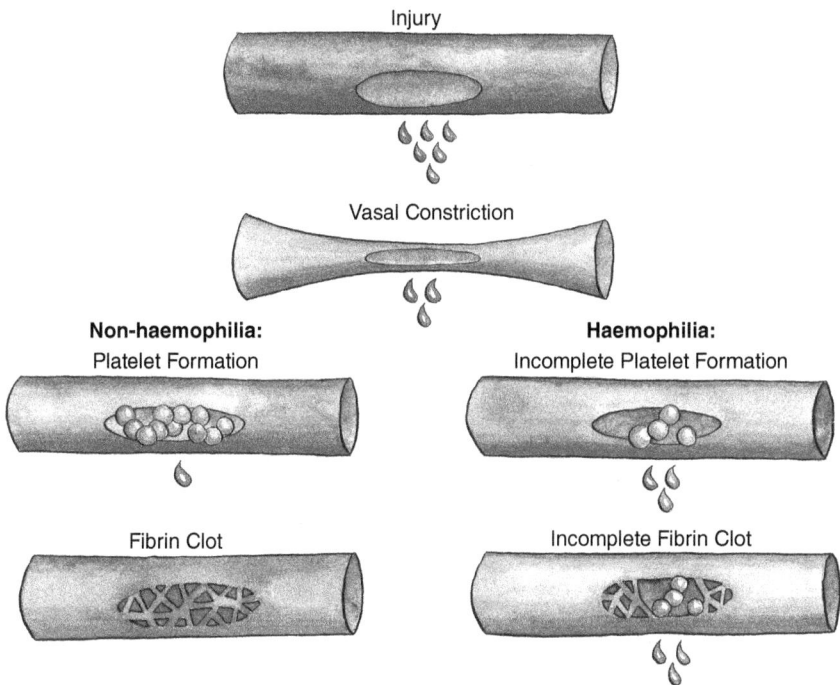

Figure 4.1 A representation of the clotting process.

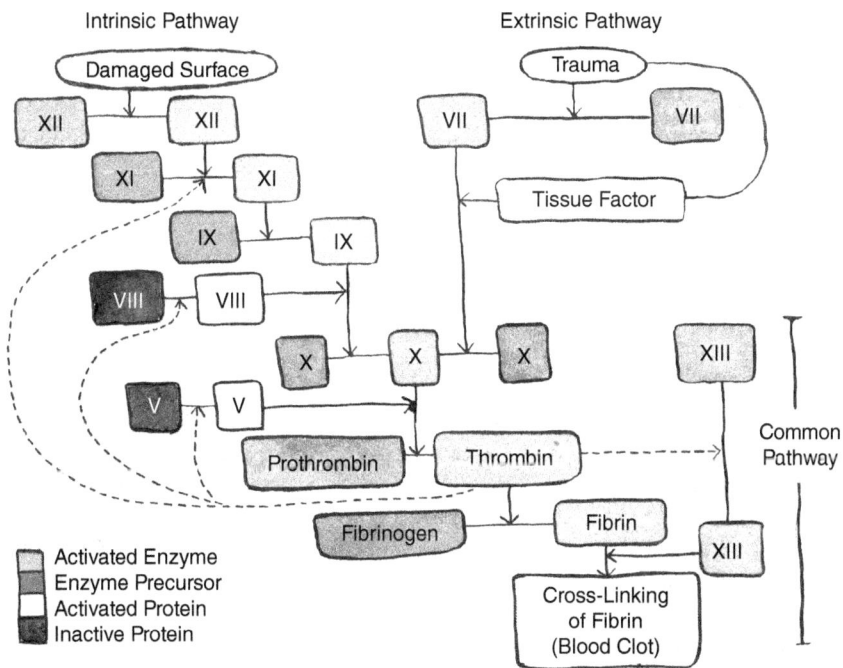

Figure 4.2 Complexity of the clotting cascade.

When a blood vessel is injured, the walls of the blood vessel contract to limit the flow of blood to the damaged area. Then, small blood cells called platelets stick to the site of injury and spread along the surface of the blood vessel to stop the bleeding. At the same time, chemical signals are released from small sacs inside the platelets that attract other cells to the area and make them clump together to form what is called a platelet plug. On the surface of these activated platelets, many different clotting factors work together in a series of complex chemical reactions (known as the coagulation cascade) to form a fibrin clot. The clot acts like a mesh to stop the bleeding. Coagulation factors circulate in the blood in an inactive form. When a blood vessel is injured, the coagulation cascade is initiated and each coagulation factor is activated in a specific order to lead to the formation of the blood clot. (*Inherited Bleeding Disorders. © WFH 2014. http://elearning.wfh.org/elearning-centres/ inherited-bleeding-disorders/#clotting_process*)

Treatment with clotting factor replacement products, especially home treatment, produced a radically new haemophilia: a haemophilia where many ordinary everyday activities were possible and where someone with severe haemophilia could realistically expect an average life span. In the better off countries of the world, including New Zealand, the time between the advent of readily available, effective treatment, and the realisation that there was HIV in some of these treatment products is often referred to as 'the golden age'. In most countries, it was less than two decades. In New Zealand, it began in the late 1960s and ended with the first diagnosis of treatment-related HIV in 1984. Also in 1984, the gene for FVIII was characterised and cloned (see Figure 4.3). It was this genetic research that led to the development of recombinant clotting factor products not made from blood.

Recombinant clotting factor

Polymerase chain reaction (PCR) techniques in molecular biology allow the amplification of single copies of small pieces of DNA, and enable the analyses that led to finding those genes on the X chromosome that control factors VIII and IX. PCR has many uses, such as in forensics, in the study of connections between groups of humans and/or animals, as well as in the diagnosis of genetic disorders, and, in this case, in opening the door to new treatment for haemophilia. In the production of haemophilia products, PCR is used to produce synthetic clotting factor that does not rely on animal or human tissue. It took a few more years for the factor IX gene to be characterised, and in 1992 and 1997 respectively the first recombinant products for FVIII and FIX became available (WFH 2015).

Recombinant products were initially donated, like those given to Luke who was one of the first little boys in New Zealand to be treated by this product. The kind of haemophilia that Luke had was not only able to be

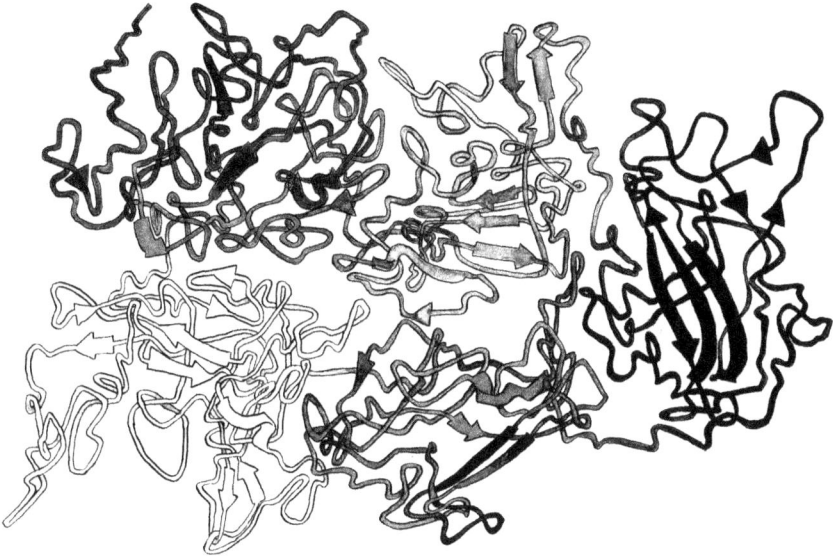

Figure 4.3 Representation of factor VIII gene.

treated very well but, unlike that of the children diagnosed even a year earlier, it was not the kind of haemophilia where parents had to be worried about hepatitis C. The new worry was about continuity of supply and cost. The network of care had gained a new participant class: multinational pharmaceutical companies. This technology involved the parents in a direct relationship with the pharmaceutical company and with the Department (later Ministry) of Health and their haemophilia treatment centre to maintain the supply of this product.

The transformation of most people with haemophilia from recipients of products manufactured from the scarce resource of donated blood to consumers of recombinant products manufactured and sold by multinational companies did not go unnoticed by members of the community. One mother, Win, told us a story in 2006 (Park and York 2008, 20–21). It concerned her 13-year-old son whose haematologist had wanted him to transfer to a recombinant product, manufactured by a different company, about 18 months earlier. This boy had heard that other children had been offered inducements such as cell phones and goody bags to change companies, so he asked what was in it for him. The haematologist was nonplussed, but when the boy explained, he supposed he 'might run to a can of Coke and a bag of chips', and his young patient was quite satisfied, to Win's amusement. Win explained that her son had been a [drug company name] kid since he was four years old, 'when they first introduced the six months free to get you hooked on it'. Community members were well aware that the multinational companies were vying for their business and that they,

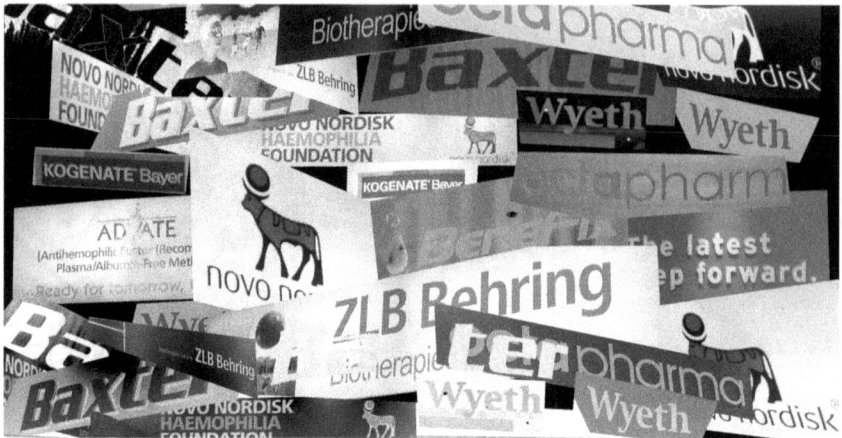

Figure 4.4 Signs of pharmaceuticalisation at WHF congress.

and then PHARMAC when it began purchasing, had choices. However, they also knew that these were not free choices in a perfect market. Win explained that she was concerned that her son might develop inhibitors if he used a new product and that if he did, they would not be able to go back to their original company (see Figure 4.4).

Several participants discussed this new network of care in terms of the drug companies' first duty being to their shareholders and the need to make a profit, but tempered this by recognising the need for profits for investment in improved treatment products. That New Zealand is a small and distant market raised fears about continuity of supply: a trade war, manufacturing problems, or transport issues could interrupt supply. The cost of products in light of funding constraints on the national health budget also induced a sense of vulnerability. Those who discussed such matters thought that there was a difficult balance for PHARMAC in getting the lowest price for the products it bought for the haemophilia community without making the New Zealand market unattractive to these large multinational companies.

On demand and prophylaxis at home and elsewhere

At first, treatment products were used to stop bleeds by increasing the level of clotting factor after a bleed was underway. Under this regimen, several treatments might be needed after a bleed to create a stable clot as the infused clotting factor has a relatively short half-life. The object is to achieve a sufficiently high and consistent enough factor level to allow a clot to form and be maintained. This treatment on demand is now used mainly by people with mild to moderate haemophilia, for some adults with severe haemophilia who are not so prone to bleeds, and for people with severe haemophilia using prophylaxis who need some additional replacement therapy.

Many people in New Zealand took up the option of treating themselves or their children at home from the 1980s on and, where haemophilia was severe, adopting prophylaxis from the 1990s (Coopers and Lybrand 1995). Internationally, prophylaxis was used sporadically by certain physicians from 1950, but it was not routinely in use until the 1990s.

Prophylaxis involves the regular (usually two to three times a week) administration of clotting factor replacement therapy to maintain factor levels consistently high enough to completely prevent the spontaneous bleeds that typify most severe and some moderate haemophilia. It made a huge difference to people's lives, as a mother of a preschooler who had just switched to prophylactic treatment explained in 1995:

> I did [preschool] by correspondence for four-and-a-half years and then tried kindy [kindergarten] but he missed one out of [every] three sessions with bleeds. Now he's on prophylaxis he's missed no sessions.

The social and educational benefits, as well as pain minimisation, are obvious in this example as in June's earlier story. Additionally, for the first time since her son was born, this mother had some time to herself while he went to morning kindergarten. The mother of a slightly older boy explained how prophylaxis had improved her son's general health.

> He was always tired and he always grizzled. And yet there wouldn't be anything obviously wrong except that he had 15 or 20 bruises on his body, but he didn't have any joint bleeds. That was all he was treated for until the prophylaxis [treatment] started. But yeah, he's a different child.
> (Mother of a 5-year-old with severe haemophilia)

Like all treatment for haemophilia, prophylaxis was and is available only in well-off countries with state-funded health care, or to the wealthy in other countries. In recent years, research from pharmaceutical companies has gone into extending the half-life of the replacement products in order to reduce the frequency of prophylactic treatment. Long-acting treatments are one of the hopes for the future for people with haemophilia.

Supply: health services as technology

When we first began our research, we discovered that certain areas of New Zealand at particular times did not have enough treatment product for people with haemophilia for everyday living. The consequences ranged from the inconvenient—keeping the boys indoors for a couple of days until supply was resumed, to the dramatic—delaying urgent surgery until more product could be located. These shortages of product were usually the result of the way the regional blood services were organised (NBTSAC 1994). At this time, with a regionalised blood service, the amount of haemophilia treatment product available in a region was related to the 'bleed rate' of that local population, i.e., the amount of blood that had been donated from that particular region. The region's donations were sent off to Australia to be fractionated and returned as replacement therapy. As a consequence, the amount of product available was not related to the numbers of people with haemophilia who lived in the region but to how generous the people in that area had been in donating blood.

Haematologists tried to overcome these created shortages in informal ways by moving product across regions' borders. They and others also agitated for a national blood service. This was achieved in 1998 with the formation of the New Zealand Blood Service as a statutory corporation with the Ministers of Health and Finance as shareholders, and greatly assisted. However, the regional organisation of the health services that has prevailed for most of the last 30 years, created another level of problems. By 2006, with a national New Zealand Blood Service and recombinant products purchased centrally by PHARMAC, the problem of uneven access was not so much over the absolute availability of treatment products, but over the mismatch between the district health board's funding and the costs of haemophilia care in each area. The networks of care were themselves producing inefficiencies and inequalities in treatment, but how this happened changed over time.

There is never enough money in the government's health budget to provide for all the nation's health needs. Preventative services have to vie with curative services, public health with personal health, common diseases with rare and expensive ones, and so on. When budget-holding for health is regionalised, rare, expensive conditions like haemophilia can devastate a region's budget. To make matters worse, as an inherited condition, haemophilia tends to clump if families are residentially stable. A large extended family with haemophilia in a small district health board area creates financial headaches, as do a large cohort of adolescent boys, the heaviest users of treatment products. The organisational technology that ultimately has addressed this problem is the National Haemophilia Management Group [NHMG], which manages the haemophilia budget and the supply of treatment products nationally in a way that is responsive to the actual treatment needs of the haemophilia population wherever they are in New Zealand. Boys no longer need to be shut indoors so that they do not hurt themselves by falling off their bikes until more product is released in the region.

This more certain supply raises a new topic in haemophilia discussions: 'What are the limits?' Virtually everyone in the haemophilia community knows that treatment is expensive. There are debates about whether, for example, young men especially, should be using this publicly-funded product so that they can pursue somewhat dangerous sports. The wider community and particular couples also discuss whether, after having one or two boys with haemophilia, couples should contemplate having any more. In 2003, these discussions about costs, efficacy, and use of treatment were carried on more publicly in the pages of the *New Zealand Medical Journal*

(Carnahan 2003; Faed 2003; Harper *et al.* 2003). In this debate, the concept of partnerships in care between people with haemophilia, their organisation, and the haematology specialists was part of the solution for effective and responsible treatment of haemophilia.

The new technologies of care, a national blood and recombinant product service combined with a national haemophilia service, no longer impose restraints as directly as did absolute shortages. But they have given rise to a new regimen of self-management based on a sense of moral commitment to the wider community: not using too much of the national health resource, or the haemophilia dollar. While the 'self-managing citizen' is central to neoliberal political philosophy (Rose 2006; Trnka 2017, 31), this version of it, we suggest, is also linked to arcadian ideals of having enough as a community because each person or family ideally moderates their wants in the interest of the common good.

Networks of collaborative care

Because haemophilia is a lifelong and intergenerational condition that may affect several branches of an extended family, strong and knowledgeable intrafamilial networks of care may build up over time. Where the haemophilia specialist workforce is stable, as it has been in many parts of New Zealand, relations between patients, families, and health workers are marked by mutual respect. Expert patients are recognised by experienced doctors. The wife of a man with haemophilia reported to us the words of her haematologist that were addressed to a junior doctor: 'Listen to Mrs. Beeson, she has been treating her husband for 30 years'. This 'partnership of care' approach was widespread, although not universal, at all periods of our research.

These existing characteristics of the networks of care provide a context within which new electronic communication devices have found a place in treatment (see Jutel 2011). For many years, it was a struggle for people with haemophilia or their parents to keep track of treatment details in paper diaries, along with the batch numbers of their products, bleeding episodes and other relevant incidents. The advent of electronic devices and inventive Apps allow people with haemophilia to record this information quickly. These data can be instantly transmitted to their treatment centre and possibly to a pharmaceutical company or research trial and used by the person with haemophilia or their parents. Studies of such technologies overseas report that the electronic communication is usually enthusiastically received and experienced as a highly superior method of keeping track of treatments and bleeds (Arnold *et al.* 2005).

Participants in New Zealand reinforce this positive reception. The relationship with the treatment centre, feeling part of the health care team, and an understanding of the benefits of close monitoring of this expensive and sometimes difficult treatment, seems to dominate the technology's reception. In addition, the experience of contaminated product in the past has alerted the haemophilia community to the importance of recording batch numbers and being very attentive to product recall. These new devices have slotted into a network of care where partnerships are the norm and they take their meaning as a technology from these pre-existing relationships. As a result, rather than surveillance being the experience, the exchange of information among the team is seen as a benefit, with convenience running a close second.

Being able to carefully monitor expiry dates themselves and thus conserve product and keep a close eye on the amount of product consumed is an aspect of good citizenship for people with haemophilia in New Zealand who are very aware that their treatment is funded through the taxes of fellow citizens and is a significant cost to the health budget (Park and York 2008). It enables close liaison with the New Zealand Blood Service to use up short-dated stock, for example. More broadly, electronic technologies, such as Facebook, Skype, and similar have strengthened biosociality in this dispersed community in New Zealand and overseas, enabling social support, information exchange and friendship within the haemophilia community, and supporting collective action. They enhance empowerment but also increase the responsibilities of individuals and the community, contributing to a positive biosociality. Adult participants frequently felt empowered to tinker independently of their doctors with their dosages, frequencies, and exercise regimes to reach the optimum balance. Biopower, in such instances, as Rabinow and Rose (2006, 200) propose, is a positive power to enhance life.

Gene therapy

> Nita (in 2005): No, if it [gene therapy] makes my baby healthy, happy, and—'well protected' is sort of the wrong word—but more like everybody else, so he can play or run or do whatever he wants, without mummy having to fear that he is going to be hurt and end up in hospital, why would you not use it?

Nita added a significant proviso: 'as long as gene therapy has been properly tested'. Nita was hopeful about gene therapy and willing to use it, but like everyone else in the community, she was dependent on the efficacy of scientific processes to ensure that this new therapy is safe, and even with that assurance was still a little apprehensive.

Understandings of gene therapy

But what exactly is gene therapy for haemophilia? From the biomedical point of view, gene therapy involves the insertion of a desired gene into a cell. It requires a vector, which in recent trials is a specially improved virus that infects humans but does not cause disease (e.g., adeno-associated virus serotype 8 (AAV8)) (NIH 2014). The virus has the relevant nonmutated gene inserted into it and, if successful, it delivers this gene into the cells it infects.

Within the haemophilia community, there were several understandings of this therapy. Especially in the early phases of our study, a few understood gene therapy as a once-and-for-all procedure carried out on an embryo to 'get rid of the bad gene instead of aborting the child', or perhaps carried out on a grown person, in which case it would provide a lifelong cure. The once-and-for-all scenario was noted by an older man who had followed gene therapy closely for decades as the initial way it had been described to him. But by the twenty-first century the 'top up' approach was what was mostly talked about. Most by then understood gene therapy as not a cure but a form of prophylactic treatment that might activate production of factor VIII or IX. At best, it might allow someone with severe haemophilia, for example, to have sufficient clotting factor to be classified as moderate or even mild. How this might happen might be through 'a jab' or a pill, or perhaps some kind of implant of genetic material that would, for a while at least, manufacture clotting protein in one's body. A few people mentioned that trials had been done on dogs and some on humans but that there were unresolved problems including some major health issues. A number talked about the virus vector that was used to introduce the 'clotting gene', two mentioning that a modified HIV virus was one of those experimented with, 'an unsettling thought, given the history of haemophilia' as Andy, a man in his thirties with haemophilia, pointed out.

Qualified acceptance

Several people expressed reservations about unintended long-term consequences of gene therapy, even if trials had been properly completed. This disquiet was often expressed in terms of gene therapy going against what was natural, or against what the body was designed to do. For example, Don had used the Internet to read up on gene therapy and he and his wife, Deb, had discussed it in some detail. Although they would consider gene therapy for a child, to them it was 'scary because it changes the molecular structure'.

Tui had heard about gene therapy only from movies and TV and although she thought that 'it doesn't sound very natural', she said that if there were 'older adults who have used it and go through it and then to hear first-hand from somebody that has been through all that, and then I might consider it'. Tui did not place as much emphasis as most others on the scientific evidence. For her, learning directly from people who have had gene therapy was the key. Tui's wish that older adults be the first to trial it was because she felt that there were too many risks for children. Older adults had already had a chance at life. This view was widespread. Several people expressed admiration for men who subjected themselves to trials of new treatments. Two men, one in his thirties and another around 60, said that they would be prepared to be part of a trial, giving a rationale that they had benefitted from others' participation in trials and they would prefer grown men rather than children put themselves at risk.

The cautious but not oppositional approach to gene therapy meant that New Zealand 'not being at the cutting edge' of gene therapy was seen as an advantage. There would be time to observe its implementation elsewhere. For genetic therapy of any kind, participants noted that there was always the possibility of what Anna described as 'science gone mad'—technologies that had the potential for good to be used for evil.

Conversations about gene therapy indicated that although nearly everyone had a degree of confidence in scientific medical trials and would not consider making a major change in treatment that had not been trialled, trials alone were not quite enough. People live with haemophilia their whole lifetime; families live with it for generations. Compared with this multigenerational time-span, trials are short-term. Gene therapy for haemophilia was part of a future-oriented economy of hope (Novas 2006), but one that was tinged with fear. This was one area in which most people were cautious about being the bold guinea pigs that Lynette had described.

Those people who had followed the fortunes of gene therapy trials for a decade or two, described this therapy as an always-distant horizon or as a ship that never comes closer, even in 2006. One mother surmised that this scepticism was a protection against disappointment. In contrast, some of the younger people or those who had only recently come in contact with haemophilia were more hopeful about its application. One of these young men was Euan. He told us in 2005 that the 'ray of sunshine on the horizon' was that gene therapy would only be necessary infrequently, compared with current prophylactic treatment, and would not be intravenous. In the wider community, 'infrequently' was variously understood. It might be once a week, once a year, or every few years. When discussing frequency, several people noted the efforts of drug companies to extend the half-life of their recombinant products and therefore reduce the frequency of injections. This was seen as more likely to eventuate in the near future than gene therapy. As well as the convenience it represented, less frequent treatments would reduce the damage caused to veins by thousands of treatments over a lifetime.

The context of acceptance

Given that many New Zealanders are opposed to the presence of genetically modified organisms, it might seem puzzling that people with haemophilia, who had been so badly affected by viruses, were prepared to contemplate and accept a genetically engineered treatment that also involved viral vectors. The 'clean green' image of New Zealand is seen by many as incompatible with genetically modified organisms. As a result of a case brought by a local authority and other groups, the Environment Court in 2015 determined that local communities have the right to control genetically modified organisms through the Resource Management Act. A strong Māori voice has been heard in many of the debates and cases relating to genetic modification. For example, Govern and Wuthnow (2004) and Scott and

Tipene-Matua (2004) both argue against a reductionist approach and for a relational approach more in consonance with Māori world views. Such a stance is authorised by recognition of the Treaty of Waitangi in the governing legislation for the bodies regulating genetic research and practice in areas such as health and agriculture.

Our research has led us to suggest that the relative openness of the haemophilia community to gene therapy, despite general valuing of what is 'natural', can be explained in part by the history of technologies of care. This community was already very familiar with recombinant clotting products. These were used to treat all of the younger people with haemophilia unless there were clinical reasons to do otherwise. HFNZ has worked with haematologists, drug companies and PHARMAC to make this possible. Recombinant products have almost completely obviated safety issues around viral contamination of clotting factor products. This routine use of a product that has been genetically engineered through PCR was highlighted by several people as significant in provoking them to rethink their previously unreflective anti-GE stance, and to make them more open to gene therapy and other new technologies, such as preimplantation genetic diagnosis [PGD]. Experience with haemophilia disposed them to do serious research and make them more open to GE (Park 2009, 181). Like Nita, they would consider all options that might make their child's life healthier and happier and have him or her more protected from bleeds. Significantly, despite concerns about being natural, no one interviewed opposed gene therapy outright on the grounds that it involved genetic modification.

Participants who discussed gene therapy, like Ursula below, remained very cautious or completely opposed to genetically modified crops, but they were prepared to consider GE for medical purposes, including for haemophilia, as long as there was careful ethical scrutiny and long-term trials. This is a group of people for whom genetic modification enables safer and less constrained lives, and because of this, gene therapy is almost familiar even before they have actually encountered it.

URSULA: I used to be totally against GM, but of course I have totally changed that view because of our situation, and if a cure could have eventually [be found] (trails off)

JULIE: So you have changed your view around this area, but what about other areas of genetic modification?

URSULA: Not in terms of crops, I think that is still dangerous, I don't like that idea at all. For medical only.

Obstacles to the introduction of gene therapy

People mentioned practical obstacles to the introduction of gene therapy, such as funding in the context of New Zealand's stretched health services. A leader in the haemophilia community warned that gene therapy would come with a price tag that was not necessarily the cost of production and distribution, but the price based on its high value to the community. Then there would be the effects of this treatment possibly replacing what are at present conventional treatment products (plasma-derived or recombinant) with consequent reduction of options and changes in cost structures. He reflected on the contrast that he had observed in the haemophilia community between worries about the safety of current blood products and the relatively relaxed approach to gene therapy, despite its experimental nature. Several people noted that gene therapy would probably involve taking immuno-suppressants to prevent rejection, and this could cause problems.

A postscript

By the time we were writing this book, gene therapy was becoming something that again seemed to be just around the corner for this community, rather than on the ever-distant far horizon described earlier. In a 2011 Editorial in *Molecular Therapy*, the Associate Journal Editor and the President of the World Federation of Hemophilia (High and Skinner 2011) commented on recent successful trials and suggested that these would have critical implications for treatment worldwide, and perhaps most especially in resource-poor countries. Successful trials with long-term beneficial effects and low levels of side effects continue to be reported. For example, one such trial with older men in London had showed sustained success in maintaining higher clotting factor levels for up to four years. This trial was being extended to younger men (NIH 2014). The community scepticism that we reported from our 2005–6 study was being replaced with a sense that gene therapy was on the verge of becoming another type of technology of treatment, but it was not the cure for haemophilia.

   Genetic technologies underlie the other aspect of technologies introduced at the beginning of the chapter, namely technologies of testing. These too take much of their meaning from their context and can be experienced as care, as giving choice, as oppression, or as a mixture of these and other possibilities.

Technologies for testing

New developments in testing technologies create new haemophilia experiences and dilemmas. Testing is used for diagnosis when there are symptoms, to pin-point the mutation, for checking carrier status, for finding out if a foetus has haemophilia. Testing may come into play at any time of life and has different implications depending on gender and life stage. For example, a little boy had unexplained bruising. After some delay, a series of tests led to the conclusion that he had severe haemophilia A. There was no known history in his family. But, as described in chapter 2, after her test the grandmother announced 'I am your time bomb' accepting diagnosis and responsibility at the same time. Before genetic testing was available, there would have been no reason for the grandmother to have conceptualised herself as a time bomb implicated in her grandson's haemophilia. Rather, new mutations in the mother or son may have been suspected.

Carriers fall into two categories with unequal access to knowledge of their carrier status. Daughters of men with haemophilia can grow up always knowing that they carry haemophilia if someone explains transmission to them. The daughters of women carriers, and their parents and caregivers, are in a much more contested space, especially if they are asymptomatic. Only a genetic test can give them a definitive diagnosis. While a low factor level will suggest carrier status in a woman, a normal level does not rule it out. For asymptomatic suspected carrier women, confirmation of their status—other than by giving birth to a boy with haemophilia—is by genetic analysis.

Contemporary genetic testing for haemophilia has gone hand-in-hand with treatment with recombinant products: both are dependent on the isolation and characterisation of the genes involved, and these in turn were dependent on research in molecular genetics and the sequencing of the human genome (Pruthi 2005). At present, despite 30 per cent of haemophilia being sporadic, prospective population screening is not carried out due to the condition's rarity. Genetic testing in this chapter therefore refers to testing in particular families where there is suspected or confirmed haemophilia.

As more research has been done on the genes for factor VIII and IX, the specific and varied mutations that give rise to haemophilia and their particular effects have become better understood. However, a small percentage of cases of haemophilia still have unidentified mutations (Pruthi 2005). In the majority of cases where the mutations are identified, direct genetic testing has specific advantages in addition to confirming a diagnosis. Some mutations are more likely to produce inhibitors to treatment products and this provides important knowledge for treatment strategies. Genetic analysis in the case of a carrier woman with no known family history of haemophilia can provide an indication of severity levels for any boys she may have, as different mutations give rise to different severity levels. Genetic analysis in men with haemophilia provides a foundation for efficient testing of any female relatives and for prenatal tests. Prenatal tests can provide the basis for the management of birth and postnatal care (Pruthi 2005), although, in New Zealand, the expected standard of care is that all births by carrier women are treated as if the baby has haemophilia, so testing is more usually done after the birth. All of these beneficial effects of genetic technologies and the familiarity of the tests themselves mean that in a society like New Zealand, haemophilia is not usually imagined as a family weakness, punishment, or a curse but quite specifically as a genetic condition. Testing for it can appear to be quite routine: just 'a little test' as one mother related.

Like the clotting time and factor level assays before them, genetic tests for boys and men with haemophilia were routinely done and assimilated into haemophilia care as an advance, which gave more knowledge and certainty about severity and tendency toward inhibitors. Given that what was being tested and discussed was inheritable, one might expect it to lead to a discussion of men passing haemophilia on, but this was not the case. However, in the contexts of prenatal and carrier testing, the situation was very different. Discussion and debate about reproduction abounded, potential carriers might be transformed into women with haemophilia, and new dilemmas were created.

Testing for carriers

Carrier testing of girls and young women raised different ideas held by members of the community about parenting, child development, and everyday ethics. The debates and actions of parents and young women made visible ethical principles, which differentially valued autonomy and relatedness, the personal and the societal, and can be analysed through what Mol (2008) called the logics of choice and care.

The goals of parents whose daughters were potential carriers were to provide age-appropriate understandings, acceptance of possible carrier status, and practical knowledge about managing this. Two seven-year olds, playing together at a summer haemophilia camp exemplified this aspiration well. One little girl said to her friend: 'Well, I'm a carrier of haemophilia and that means that if I have boys they might have haemophilia'. Her friend said, 'Is that mild or moderate?' and they just carried on playing. However, it was apparent that some cousins or haemophilia camp friends knew their carrier status and others did not.

Parents often drew attention to the parallel that they saw with children's knowledge about being adopted. Many wished that their girls could grow up 'always knowing' their status. In caring for their children, and giving them the best chance to integrate an understanding of haemophilia into their development of self, many parents wanted their girls to know whether they were carriers before adolescence—although the exact timing was debated. Parents also pointed out that nonobligate carrier daughters were not always in a position to learn much about what haemophilia was through their everyday observations either, unless they had affected brothers, cousins or maternal uncles nearby.

Care for their daughters led some parents to have their children tested early and then choose the appropriate time to let them know, as Murray and Mary suggested in 2006. They particularly wanted to avoid springing the news of her carrier status on a daughter who was already experiencing the struggles of adolescence. In addition, they did not want to wait until their daughter had an accident or had to have dentistry or surgery to find out that she had bleeding problems:

MURRAY: I think it [carrier testing of young girls] is important in so far as you take away the element of surprise, you are aware of it the whole time. So if you are aware of something, and perhaps information that will crop up along the way, like you'll put it in the back of your memory, rather than being dropped in it at the last minute, when you are not really educated about the whole deal.

MARIE: I agree with carrier testing, and I reckon it should be done as soon as possible, before they are teenagers, you know the whole issue of them only having factor VIII level tested as an indicator, and then having it confirmed with genetic testing later on, when they are able to give consent, at 15 or 16. To me that is just a little bit late. Because they are dealing with a whole lot of other issues and to have it sprung on them, 'Yes, you are a carrier', you know!

MURRAY: It's a terrible time anyway.

MARIE: And, who knows, hopefully not, they might get pregnant when they are only 13 or something!

This couple thought that somewhere around 11–13 years, or earlier, was a good time to make sure their daughter understood what being a carrier entailed. Whether couples favoured learning about carrier status in early childhood or in the midteenage years, their approaches to informing their daughters were very different from some earlier generations. One middle-aged woman told us during a chat in 1995, that on the evening before her wedding she was sat down by her parents and told that she was a carrier of haemophilia. Like other women of her generation she was determined that her daughters would not have to face such an ill-timed revelation about their status.

Debate about the best age for carrier testing was one time we heard a heated exchange about a personal matter at a HFNZ occasion. Foundation members quite frequently debated business matters with some heat, but for what are seen as individual and moral issues, such as prenatal testing, family planning and so on, usually people resort to the value of 'What's right for the family is what's right', to mediate differences of opinion and practice. New Zealand guidelines for carrier testing were under discussion at an AGM. One member argued strongly, in line with the guidelines, that genetic testing of potential carrier girls should be delayed until the girls were of an age to consent, i.e., 16 years. Her argument made use of the concepts of autonomy and choice in relation to the girl. On hearing this, the husband of a carrier woman made the point that if his daughter were a carrier he would want to consider carefully whether to have any more children who carried haemophilia. He was also using the concept of choice, but it was his own choice that was at issue because of his concern about the morality of bringing more children with haemophilia into the world, given the demands on the health system that they make.

The reasons offered by other men who did not want to have (more) carrier daughters included care for their immediate family as well as a sense of citizenship. They explained that haemophilia in their daughters' future sons was a difficult condition for their girls to cope with and painful and difficult for their grandsons. It was also an expensive charge on their fellow citizens.

In the meeting, this view was disputed by the first speaker noted above, and the rights of the child to privacy and autonomy were championed by a small but adamant group who argued that potential carriers could still be brought up with the knowledge that they might be carriers and what this entailed, but they should be able to choose for themselves, as adults, to be tested. This was a minority view and it was not met with in interviews or other venues, but it was passionately held by the group at the meeting. This view coincided with that of those creating and promulgating the New Zealand guidelines (National Advisory Committee on Health and Disability 2003).

In our research with the girls and young women themselves, we found arguments or practices both for and against these positions. For example, one young woman had a carrier test done at age 18 and did not tell her parents. They had encouraged her to be tested earlier, but she had not wanted this. In another instance, after hearing the debate about carrier testing guidelines, a mother confided to us that she had had her daughter tested when she was very young and she wondered whether her daughter, Natasha, resented this. On the contrary, her daughter who was also a participant, but interviewed in another town by a different member of the research team with no mother around, was happy that she had always known.[1] Natasha told us:

> My point of view is, I think, 'the earlier the better', you know. The more you grow up with it and it's accepted, it does become something you just get on with, and it's just what it is and you just deal with, you know, rather than, all of a sudden going, 'Oh my God, is that what it is' and, yeah, the earlier the better.

Despite always knowing her status, she said it was only when she had begun thinking about having children in her early twenties that she really began 'identifying as a carrier' and seriously considering the implications (Park and York 2008, 31).

From our interviews and workshops, we discovered that there were varied clinical practices relating to genetic testing of carriers without bleeding problems around the country, and even within clinics: everything from testing at birth, to strict adherence to not testing until the girl reached the age of consent. The parents of the three female foetuses carrying haemophilia who were born in Auckland between 1989 and 1999 knew their daughter's status before birth (Park 2005, 100). Other parents told us that they found out shortly after their baby was born through cord blood tests.

A preference for early testing of girls is supported by Ross's (1997) work on perspectives of carriers. 'Steps for Living' (NHF 2018b) discusses the advantages of early testing of possible carriers both in terms of safety and appropriate knowledge. Nonetheless, reviews of international guidelines for genetic testing (Hogben and Boddington 2006) and an article on genetic testing for haemophilia by Mayo Clinic specialist, Pruthi (2005), report that the usual recommendation for carriers is to delay testing until the age of majority or until the child is competent to consent.[2] This is in line with New Zealand discussions also (Ministry of Health 1998; P. Malpas *pers. comm.* 2009). However, the report on genetic testing by the National Advisory Committee on Health and Disability (2003) points out that parents have the legal right to consent on their child's behalf although doctors may contest this. Two different but overlapping networks of care have come to different conclusions about carrier testing.

Carrier testing of children is recognised as a complex issue in bioethics discourse. Based on his review of international and United Kingdom guidelines, Shenfield (2002, 271) concluded that there 'should be a presumption against testing young children for carrier status'. However, if a young person understands the implications and clearly consents, their informed choice to test or not should be respected. With regard to the father who would like to have his daughter tested to make choices about subsequent children, Shenfield (2002, 270) summarises the bioethical consensus as: 'children should not generally be used as a means for others to attain their goals'. Yet children are a means for their parents to attain their goals: intrinsically, the goal of becoming a parent (Park 2005). The guiding principle in these bioethical considerations is the best interests of the child. Therefore, genetic testing of symptomatic children or children who may benefit from preventive treatment is supported (Shenfield 2002, 271).

Embryonic carriers

The availability of PGD has prompted some young carrier women to discuss carriers in relation to selection of embryos for implantation. This topic was raised during a Young Woman's Workshop during our last field phase. Hannah talked to Deon about it afterwards.

> Hannah: There was the screening process itself [as part of PGD]. We had a few sessions with how they won't test girls [female embryos] and how that decision is left up to the next generation whether or not they want to go through the process again. We thought that that was a bit bizarre ... that you can screen boys to see if they have the haemophilia gene but you don't screen girls ... We thought, if you can have a carrier girl or a noncarrier girl, why would you not have a noncarrier girl, you know? It's the same as getting the haemophilia gene out, which is what you are doing by having a boy who doesn't have haemophilia. And, you know, 'because it doesn't directly impact on their lives' you say, 'you can't do that', which was a bit bizarre, but, hey, I'm sure they'll wrinkle it out and realise, see sense, hopefully. (Park and York 2008, 30)

Other young women agreed with Hannah's sentiments. They were aware of the 'soft' eugenic effects of individuals selecting against a male embryo with haemophilia and did not see that selecting against female carriers was morally any different because it would save pain and suffering over generations and remove the burden of being a carrier from the girl. As they saw it, not selecting was simply postponing the problem and transferring burdens to a subsequent generation. Sue echoed Hannah's views, and said: 'it's not considered a serious condition just to be a carrier ... I feel that if you can actually stop it being passed on ... why wouldn't you? It's an expensive condition to treat, apparently the most expensive' (Park and York 2008, 35).

Sue's disagreement with the idea that being a carrier was 'not serious', and Natasha's sense of 'identifying as a carrier' challenge the results of the discourse analysis of testing guidelines from Canada, the United Kingdom, and the United States, carried out by Hogben and Boddington (2006). These authors contrast predictive testing of children for later onset genetic disorders with carrier testing. They conclude that for the creators of guidelines, carrier testing is construed as less serious, limited to the reproductive domain, and therefore of concern to others rather than self, and not core self-knowledge. As a result, they suggest, carrier testing of children is likely to be more permissible, as the perception is of minimal risk. Sue contested the view that carrier status was not a serious matter for women and girls, and Natasha found it was an important part of her identity.

Identity, care, and choice

Because carrier testing is not deemed necessary for treatment of most young girls, in New Zealand, the social and psychological reasons for having tests done early are trumped by the cultural, often understood as ethical, values of individual privacy, consent, and individual choice, which are enshrined in testing guidelines. As our research shows, at least some potential carriers take their status in relation to haemophilia very seriously, and would like to have always known about what to them is an important matter. Thus, the social technology of carrier testing contributes to a hierarchy of differential belonging in the haemophilia community: not being a carrier, versus being a carrier, versus having haemophilia. This is in accord with the arguments of Heath, Rapp, and Taussig (2007) about the increasing geneticisation of individual and collective identity, and provides a compelling example of the contested biopolitics surrounding genetic testing.

As Hogben and Boddington's (2006) research suggested, carrier status is often presumed to be chiefly relevant to a woman's reproductive life and is about whether they have the possibility of passing on the condition to any sons and daughters. Nevertheless, as our research findings show, this is far from a simple technical issue of 'reproductive risk'. For many women, those around them and their (potential) partners, it is deeply meaningful. Natasha spoke of 'identifying as a carrier' and other participants concurred. This process of identifying was part of Natasha's thinking about having children and, simultaneously, was an aspect of her personal identity.

Our discussions with parents indicate that many of them recognise this and try to build it into their daughters' development.

The availability of a precise genetic test to confirm carrier status leads young women and their parents to make morally charged choices in contexts where not making choices is no longer an option. People within the haemophilia community come to different resolutions of the dilemma. People most closely associated with haemophilia tend to suggest that early testing of these girls is preferable so that they can healthily integrate the knowledge provided by the tests into their lives. However, as the debate at the AGM showed, this view is not universally held even by members of the community and tends to contradict the prevailing views put forward in international and New Zealand guidelines by ethicists and clinical geneticists.

Both groups have 'the best interests of the child' at heart. But some also think about other family members and 'the good of society'. In some cases, we suggest that these best interests are upheld in terms of a logic of care, i.e., caring for the psychological development of the child, especially where carrier status is seen as important self-knowledge for the girl; caring for future generations and for fellow citizens. In other cases, the emphasis is on a logic of choice, i.e., the child's eventual autonomy and right to choose. Here, carrier status is seen as a somewhat peripheral issue, of more interest to a later phase in a girl's life and to reproduction. As noted above, however, parents of children with haemophilia do not all fall into the first group, but some adopt a rights-based logic of choice approach, as do most of the bioethical experts. However, both positions are promulgated in good faith as ways of caring for vulnerable persons who, at an early stage of their lives, are not able to care or choose for themselves.

Testing the yet-to-be-born

In 1960, a group of researchers in Copenhagen reported a 'medical breakthrough' with special relevance for people with haemophilia. They had used amniocentesis to ascertain the sex of a foetus of a woman who carried haemophilia. Finding that the foetus was male, they had performed an abortion to prevent the birth of a boy with [a 50 per cent chance of having] haemophilia (Cowan 1994, 37, insertion by present authors). The woman in question figured in the reporting only as a background figure. In later articles in scientific journals about the development of prenatal testing, the pioneers and protagonists are also scientists and doctors. The names of the women are not memorialised. But women, their partners and their embryos, foetuses or babies were there all along, appearing in the journals as cases, as sources of material to be tested, and as bearers of risk of genetic and chromosomal conditions.

Scholars have analysed several overlapping discourses of genetic testing (Rapp 1991, 1993), and have pointed to the effects for all women. Rothman points out that women's dilemmas about testing tend to be medicalised and trivialised by being 'couched in the language of anxiety'. Yet when these same issues are debated by ethicists or lawyers they are hailed as 'great moral issues of our time' (Rothman 1994, 268). While recognising that prenatal testing can cause suffering for the women and men involved, we suggest that this emotional work should not obscure the ethical work of ordinary women and men in moral decision-making. They also address major moral issues and shape future contexts, alongside bioethicists and law-makers.

In 1960, the scientists were looking in the amniotic fluid for the presence of Barr bodies, discovered in 1949, which signalled female sex. By 1955, scientists had discovered that they could be detected in amniotic fluid. Cowan (1994) describes the next 15 years as a developmental stage for amniocentesis when its potential for detecting foetal characteristics other than sex was realised. Techniques that allowed the successful culturing of cells from the amniotic fluid and karyotyping chromosomes extended the use of amniocentesis. By the mid-1970s, amniocentesis had become an established technique to be offered to a much wider range of pregnant women, including older women who were at greater risk of chromosomal abnormalities in their foetuses, as well as women carriers of inherited conditions. Prenatal testing became even more powerful for haemophilia when DNA analysis of the material taken at testing became widely available during the later 1980s and 1990s. Later developments included CVS, an alternative to amniocentesis that can be used earlier in pregnancy, widespread use of sonograms to guide the test procedure, and new methods of analysis.

Prenatal tests and prenatal imaging change the experience of pregnancy even for women who do not use them. Rothman (1994) entitled her work 'The Tentative Pregnancy'. This is a pregnancy whose continuation is reliant on the outcome of medical tests, and whose reality is confirmed not by internal feelings of quickening but by ultrasound (Taylor 2000) or other technologies. As treatment for people with haemophilia became more effective and safer, and prenatal testing became more widely available, decision dilemmas intensified for women and their husbands or partners. Should they take the test and 'what to do with the results?' For families with known haemophilia in Aotearoa New Zealand, having a child with haemophilia was now undertaken in the context of genetic technologies and considerable soul-searching. These were indeed new kinds of pregnancies. The new networks of care and new technologies configured new frameworks of choice, opening up new landscapes for moral pioneering. The technologies are far from value neutral (Latour 2002).

Cultural contexts

Decisions to have or not to have a child in Aotearoa New Zealand are made within a widespread cultural understanding that young adults, especially young women, will become parents (Park and Strookappe 1996, 53). Although these expectations are less compelling in the twenty-first century, having children is often part of attaining adulthood and is widely seen as a 'natural' stage of the life course. Some women in the first phase of our study, thinking they should not have children, said they wondered what they would do and be if they could not have children of their own. One young woman told us that she 'would do everything possible to have her own [biological] children' (Park and Strookappe 1996, 54). Thus decisions, which may not be conscious, were made in a context where having biological children was the usual expectation. Cameron's analysis of interviews with New Zealanders suggested that a cultural emphasis on childbirth as a biological imperative is stronger for women than men and the 'urge', perceived as natural or biological, to have children may be felt very strongly (Cameron 1990, 48). This is the cultural context within which New Zealand parents with haemophilia in their families make decisions about having children.

Families with known histories of severe or moderate haemophilia may be referred for genetic counselling. Counselling may involve discussion about testing and termination of affected pregnancies. Dixon, Winship, and Webster (1995, 11) noted in their report on priorities for New Zealand services, 'The implications [of genetic testing] for health care services are obvious, although "individual choice" with respect to diagnosis, treatment or prevention should remain paramount'. We do not have the precise figures to estimate the difference that the introduction of prenatal testing has made to the size of the haemophilia community in New Zealand. Work on this issue from an earlier period in Sweden by Ljung, Kling, and Tedgård (1995) gives some indication of potential effects in that country. They estimated that the incidence of haemophilia was 68 per cent higher in Sweden in the 1990s than in the 1970s, but that it would be a further 40 per cent higher were it not for effective prenatal diagnosis and genetic counselling. All we can say for New Zealand is that the number of births of children with haemophilia between 1989 and 2009 was steady at around eight per year (Chantel Lauzon, *pers. comm.* 2014).

Prenatal tests for haemophilia in Aotearoa New Zealand

Most women who participated in our research were aware of prenatal testing and had a range of deeply felt experiences and views on the subject. However, the uptake of the tests was low, although our numbers are not as exact as we would like. The most frequently used test in New Zealand is CVS, used since 1989 (Van de Water *et al.* 1991). In the following decade, the number of tests per year ranged from zero to three, with a total of 18 pregnancies involved. Three male foetuses with haemophilia were terminated, all before 1994. Subsequently, no male foetuses had haemophilia and no females were terminated (E. Berry *pers. comm.* 1999). In that period, 79 babies diagnosed with haemophilia A and B were born, indicating a relatively low uptake of testing.

By 2005–6 when our third update study was conducted, debate about the new technology of preimplantation genetic diagnosis (PGD) dominated discussions about reproductive technologies. PGD involves DNA analysis of a single cell of *in vitro* fertilised (IVF) embryos when the embryos are a few days old, and the implantation of only those embryos that are female or male without haemophilia. PGD had recently been permitted by an act of Parliament (Human Assisted Reproductive Technology Act 2004), and during this research period the government recognised haemophilia as one of the genetic conditions for which two cycles of PGD would be publicly funded. The NHMG funds two cycles of PGD per year in addition to standard government funding (*pers. comm.* Mary Brasser, Haemophilia Nurse Specialist 2018). Although when first hearing of PGD, people were often quite enthusiastic because it allows for having a baby without haemophilia without the need for abortion, that enthusiasm sometimes waned as couples learned about the challenges of IVF, the destruction of embryos, and the relatively low chances of success in any one cycle (see Franklin and Roberts [2006] for research into PGD in Britain).

Information on the extent to which prenatal testing was used proved more difficult to obtain for the decade from 2000, despite the good efforts of HFNZ. We have information from only one of the two genetics testing centres: Christchurch, obtained by HFNZ in 2013. The Auckland data were not made available but staff at the Auckland Haemophilia Centre believe there were very few prenatal tests and none in recent years. During this decade, four prenatal tests were performed in Christchurch, including two tests for the same woman in different pregnancies. Both of these pregnancies were carried to term. We do not know the outcome of the other two tests.

The New Zealand Organisation for Rare Disorders (NZORD) reported the national figures for PGD during the seven years from its introduction in June 2006 until June 2013 (Forman and Baddeley 2013). Five haemophilia A carrier patients had had 10 cycles of PGD in total and one pregnancy had resulted. One of the four women whose PGD did not result in a baby subsequently had the two prenatal tests and two successful pregnancies noted above. No haemophilia B patients had undergone PGD in New Zealand by 2013, but one haemophilia B carrier had had successful outcomes from PGD in Australia. Since 2013, three women have had PGD in Auckland with one pregnancy carried to term. It is possible that more women and couples may have used these services were they more freely available and waiting lists shorter.

During the decade from 2000 to 2009, 81 babies were born with haemophilia A or B, a figure very similar to the decade before. It appears therefore that although both prenatal testing and PGD were used by members of the haemophilia community, they were not used frequently and the number of births of babies with haemophilia have been quite constant. Despite this relatively low use, the availability of these technologies has forever changed the context of having babies for people who may pass on haemophilia.

Deliberations about testing

In the 1994–5 research period, most women saw such a strong link between taking a prenatal test, a positive result, and terminating the pregnancy that they did not want to test. Opposition to abortion was seldom on religious grounds. More frequently, the value was that with children 'you took what you got' (Park and Strookappe 1996, 62). This was not only a counsel of acceptance. It included the idea that each child was to be valued, not tinkered with. Importantly for parents who already had children was: 'What message are you giving to a child with haemophilia if you abort the next?' (Park 2005, 100). 'And what message does it send to men with haemophilia?' (Park and York 2008, 36).

Testing

The minority of women or couples who had had a prenatal test did so mainly for two reasons: to prepare themselves for having a child with or without haemophilia, or to help them decide whether or not to terminate the pregnancy. Women and their partners spoke of the difficulties of deciding to test and the enormous relief when they found out their foetus was a girl, or a boy without haemophilia. Few had been planning to have a termination, no matter what the outcome.

In 1994–5, some women or couples spoke of the conflicted situation they had been placed in, having to 'agree' that they would have a termination if the result showed a boy with haemophilia when they had no intention of terminating the pregnancy. Others did not experience any direct influence from the hospital but thought that if they had the test then 'you have to do something with the results' (Park and Strookappe 1996, 63).

Some people in the 1999 and 2005–6 update studies believed that costs of life-long haemophilia treatment motivated tests being offered by the health service, and therefore women were under pressure to abort if the results were positive for haemophilia. Other women's experience had been of acceptance and support by their specialist when they had had the test to prepare themselves for their new baby, even when they had declined abortion from the outset. None of the women, however, mentioned that they were encouraged to have a prenatal test to prepare themselves for the birth of a child with possible haemophilia. This may be because best practice for carrier women giving birth is for the babe to be treated as if s/he had haemophilia until testing negative after birth, as well as because of the risks involved in testing.[3]

Vivian who had accepted the offer of testing when she unexpectedly became pregnant told us that that she had found it impossible to make a decision without the results in front of her. Women in similar positions in other countries concurred (Gates 1994, 191). However, NZHS group counselling sessions that she and we attended suggested that a pregnant woman should be well along the decision-making path before getting the test results.

A couple who had had a male foetus with haemophilia and a termination had found it so devastating that they would never undergo it again. European research has also found that women carriers and their spouses experienced terminations as very emotionally painful, and many women experienced depressive moods even years afterward (Tedgård 1998).

Not testing

Many of the people we spoke to had not had tests because they were not prepared to terminate and therefore did not wish to put their pregnancy or the baby at risk. But even avoiding a test was making a choice and entailed the responsibility of possibly having a child with haemophilia.

One couple who had a completed family of four children, two with hae-mophilia, had not had prenatal testing. The mother said that if she inad-vertently became pregnant, she would have a prenatal test, and consider termination if a male foetus had haemophilia. That way, 'I haven't destroyed anything that is healthy'.[4] Other women did not think that haemophilia alone was a sufficiently serious reason for an abortion, but if tests showed more serious health problems, e.g., spina bifida, they would consider an abortion.

Decisions about testing were not taken lightly:

> [Prenatal testing] is a really difficult one, because I find that quite a conflicting question. Part of me says, 'Yes, I should know whether I was having another haemophiliac child'. I would NOT abort, either way. I don't believe in choosing the perfect baby—'Oh, this one is not good enough, I'm going to get rid of it'. I'm sorry, that really does not sit with me at all. I think if you're given the baby then you live with what you've got. (Interview with Mary 1999)

Park has argued (2000, 2005, 2013) that stoical acceptance is an ethical approach valued in Aotearoa New Zealand and forms part of the local biology of haemophilia, influencing how people deal with pain and bleed-ing, assess risk, and manage reproduction. However, acceptance that one has haemophilia can lead to very divergent practices over the generations, especially in conjunction with the different haemophilias produced through different treatment and through family stories. Mary went on to say that she had debated the issue with her sister and her father. She described her father, as 'one of those very straight and strict [men], he said "people who have defects, genetical defects, should not breed", basically is what he said'. We had come across the same view in some of our interviews also in 1995 with a small minority of the older men. The man who expressed it most strongly and memorably was the sheep and flower breeder mentioned in chapter 3. In these cases, stoical acceptance was being resigned to not hav-ing biological children.

In making their decisions about prenatal testing or PGD from 1999 to 2006, most women or couples imagined a hopeful future for haemophilia. As a result, most people we spoke with did not regard even severe haemophilia as a life-threatening disease, and therefore, they did not take up the opportunity to use prenatal technologies for haemophilia with any great enthusiasm. For example, a woman talking about accepting a baby with haemophilia said, 'Maybe it's easy for me to say because haemophilia isn't an incredibly severe condition', and another mother of a boy with haemophilia when talking about having another baby without any prenatal testing said, 'Why wouldn't I have another baby?'. Nonetheless, even if most women would not use these technologies themselves, they thought that they should be available so that families could make their own decisions about 'what was right for them'. Our findings about the complex moral reflections that led women to take the decisions or positions that they did, concur with Williams *et al.*'s (2005) conclusions based on their work with UK women undertaking first trimester screening: these women continue to be moral pioneers even as tests become more routinised.

Men discuss testing

Many women worried about the message sent to their fathers, brothers, or sons if they had prenatal testing or terminations. In the 2005–6 update study, we focussed on talking with men with haemophilia about reproductive issues. Nine men obliged despite such matters not being a topic of everyday masculine conversation. When Deon, as interviewer, and Neil, a fifties-plus man with severe haemophilia, had a conversation about amniocentesis and CVS, they remarked on the gendered nature of such talk in the haemophilia community. Until that time, Neil had only ever discussed reproductive issues with women, and that infrequently. One was his daughter and the other a friend in the haemophilia community. We gained the strong impression that men rarely discussed the issue at all, and certainly not with other men. Deon and Neil joked about it being not as popular a topic with men as was rugby (see chapter 3), at the beginning of their conversation.

Did men feel their lives were not valued if women contemplated genetic tests and terminations? Women had voiced this concern to us although they had not discussed it with men. In contrast to the women's concerns, the men we spoke to discounted the women's concerns. The women's actions had no implications for their own lives. 'Ridiculous', one said. Nor did their own actions, for example, if they had decided not to have biological children. Although not all thought that haemophilia was serious enough for prenatal tests, terminations, or PGD, all agreed with the desirability of 'the more options the better'. One spoke of how he might not have been born if his mother had had these options, but he still favoured them. Other men in our study told us about their hopes for their daughters in regard to these reproductive technologies (Park 1990, 180).

Rather than focussing on themselves in championing the availability of choice for their daughters and other women, the men pointed to several benefits to others. They saw the benefits of choice in terms of a logic of care. Prenatal technologies would avoid children being subject to pain and suffering. Their daughters could be saved from the burden of caring for a child with haemophilia that their own mothers had borne, a care that would 'dictate so much of her life'. Testing, they thought, could also reduce the cost burden that haemophilia places on the health service: an anxiety that concerned a lot of people within the community. Thus these men with haemophilia completely ignored concerns about what testing and selective abortion or PGD 'says about our worth', and instead concentrated on future benefits to others to argue for the availability of assisted reproductive technologies for people with haemophilia (Park and York 2008, 35–38).

Making decisions

Parents or intending parents rehearsed many considerations when making reproductive decisions. As described above, an often-unarticulated desire to have children was a pervasive background. In the foreground was an evaluation of their ability to care for a (nother) child with haemophilia. This in turn was linked to their assessment of what that child's future would be like, how serious haemophilia was, how difficult it was to raise a child with haemophilia, and how capable they were. Other aspects of their ability to cope concerned their assessment of the state of their relationship with their partner, and whether support was available from extended family and/or health services.

Is haemophilia serious?

Although the majority of participants in our studies viewed haemophilia as no longer such a serious condition, this perspective was not universal. Two carrier sisters lobbying the government to implement preimplantation genetic diagnosis were reported in a newspaper article as saying they would never knowingly bring a child with severe haemophilia into the world, even with current and new treatment options, because of witnessing their father's suffering from haemophilia and its complications, and anticipating similar problems for their future sons (Wane 2004). Commenting in an interview in 2006, on one of the news stories about this family, the mother of a little boy with haemophilia, who had had no family history of the condition, said that she felt very sorry for this family with their long, sad history and she often thought: 'If only they knew what life was like now'. Even in this case where this woman disagreed with the idea that haemophilia must be avoided at all costs, she allowed for difference within the community, saying, 'but once again, they are their decisions'. These two families were both affected by severe haemophilia at the same time and in the same region of

New Zealand, but because of their different family narratives and experiences they had different haemophilias.

Considering the well-being of the child

Community members who thought haemophilia was serious enough to warrant exploring reproductive technologies included sisters who had witnessed their brothers' suffering and mothers who already had children with haemophilia, especially if they had suffered complications such as inhibitors. Pain and suffering for future sons was uppermost in the minds of those who anticipated haemophilia as a serious condition in their decision-making. Those among them who did not agree with prenatal testing or PGD faced the option of deciding not to have (more) biological children.

The parents' assessment of the quality of the child's future was not confined to haemophilia issues. A feeling that an only child would be disadvantaged was sometimes expressed. Parents of a large family explained that having some children without haemophilia in their family took the pressure and emphasis off the children with haemophilia, enabling them to have a more normal childhood. And then there was 'What message are you giving to a child with haemophilia if you abort the next?'

Looking one or two generations ahead, many people felt that new technologies of treatment might obviate the need for frequent intravenous injections, therefore the future of children and grandchildren could be quite rosy. As one particularly optimistic young parent said in 1995, 'In 20 years from now when she is going to be having a family, haemophilia might be a thing of the past'. New technologies of both testing and therapy were part of the economy of hope.

However, imagining the well-being of future children could lead to the opposite conclusion. Although only a minority of contemporary parents had adopted children, those who talked to us about it, and who had no fertility problems, had done so because they did not want to inflict pain and suffering on children or grandchildren. A parents' sense of guilt was mentioned by some and evident in the narratives of others. A woman who had had a baby with unexpected haemophilia said in 1995, 'I couldn't do that to my family again, especially to [my baby and his father]. I felt very guilty'. Men and women who came to these conclusions were usually those who had severe or moderate haemophilia in their families and who had observed a family member: father, brother, or occasionally a female relative, having serious problems with haemophilia and its complications. However, occasionally, a daughter of a man with mild haemophilia that had hardly troubled him at all might decide against having children. Both negative experiences and a lack of experience might lead to the same conclusion.

People who had had reasonably positive experiences of haemophilia tended not to see passing haemophilia on as inflicting pain and suffering on a future generation. For example, one mother described her reaction to a doctor's advice against having a baby with haemophilia: 'it's not, to me, ... a life-threatening disease. I thought no, I mean you can live with haemo. So I overrode him' (Park and Strookappe 1996, 60). Another noted that the lifestyles of her relatives with moderate haemophilia were not restricted. Therefore, she was prepared to have a child with haemophilia. She added that were it a much more severe form, she would possibly make a different decision.

And what about the good of society?

Whereas in our initial study members of the haemophilia community seldom mentioned the effects of increasing numbers of people with haemophilia on treatment services and on health expenditure, there was more consideration of these issues by the time of the update studies. HFNZ has counselled its members to think carefully about having more children and to consider the broader issues involved. Individuals also raised these issues in interviews and discussions. Yet, to terminate a foetus with a costly disorder to spare resources is described by an ethicist, Harper, as 'particularly unsavoury'. Harper advises that while attempting to prevent pain and suffering and to allow reproductive choice should be the aim of testing programmes, the consequences for children born with the disorder should also be considered, especially the evaluation of testing programmes on the basis of numbers of affected babies born (Harper 1997 in Shenfield 2002, 271). Nonetheless, constant reminders of how much treatment products cost had their own effects.

The consequences for children, noted by Harper, was a consideration for some community members, although probably not quite in the form anticipated by Harper. This consideration related more specifically to the empowerment of the haemophilia community, given the advent of PGD. In 2006 one of the young women we interviewed expressed the view that it was good to have prenatal testing and PGD but she would be very sad if so many people used these technologies and terminated affected pregnancies that the only people with haemophilia left were sporadic cases caused by new mutations. Her reasoning was based on the support and advocacy provided by HFNZ because of the long-term, multigenerational experiences of its members. Sporadic cases would all be new to haemophilia and would not be in a powerful position to provide advocacy. The use of these technologies could create a new and much less powerful haemophilia community, less able to care for its members or to work with government for a good haemophilia service (Park and York 2008). This young woman was in favour of choices being available but rather like the ethicist, Harper, for her too, choice was tempered with care for the biosocial community of people with haemophilia.

The good of the wider society could also be a reason to value the continuation of haemophilia in the community. One aspect of this is the maintenance of diversity. Some noted that if, through 'successful' genetic engineering, haemophilia and other genetic disorders were eliminated, the limits of tolerance of difference in our society would be narrowed (see also Baird, *et al.* 1995; IHC 1995). While no parents would wish haemophilia on anyone, their children with haemophilia were the characters that they were partly because of their experiences with haemophilia, and parents valued this. They suggested that raising a happy, healthy child with hae-mophilia could be a positive contribution to a more accepting attitude to disability in the community: allowing the putatively normal population the opportunity to interact with people who are full persons and who have something wrong with them: 'He's a boy first and a haemophilia second'. This discourse is by no means confined to haemophilia families but can be found in many disability communities and in disability rights debates (Oliver 1990; Shakespeare 2006; Zola 1977, 232).

Conclusion

> [It] was sort of frightening, being away from mum and dad for so long, and that was back in the days when visiting hours was two to three [o'clock]. That was it. The head nurse at three o'clock would come around and literally shove people out.
>
> (An older man reflecting on his boyhood experiences)

Technologies and networks of care have changed over the time of this research and over the memory span of our participants. These changes have produced different haemophilias, to the point now when a mother does not know whether her son has done his treatment or not, it is so quick, and parents are not visitors to be shoved out at 3 p.m. but partners in care, as are patients themselves. Embedded in the networks of care are the stories of the past and present and imagined futures. While these stories incorporate technical matters, they are not determined by them, as people create their own understanding and lived realities of haemophilia. In turn, these stories influence how people respond to and make decisions about new technologies of treatment and testing, and inform their choices and cares. One specific example is the considered response to gene therapy that several participants explained by their familiarity with recombinant treatment products.

An ethics of care completely intertwined with an ethics of choice is a marked feature of the way haemophilia is enacted in Aotearoa New Zealand. As we showed in this chapter, the foci of care differ, as do choices, but the need to preserve both care and choice is constant. Differences in choices are accommodated within the haemophilia community by a strong value of 'what's right for the family is what's right'. As one would expect in a biosocial community plucked at random from the general population because of genetic mutation, a whole spectrum of values is represented. Children and future children with or without haemophilia are a common focus of care when choices are to be made, but so too are existing men and women with haemophilia. When thinking about testing or aborting foetuses with haemophilia, for example, many women were very concerned about the message that this would send to men with haemophilia. But the men with haemophilia whose thoughts on this topic we canvassed thought that such a consideration was not relevant. They were already alive and had lives that were not just 'living haemophilia'.

Care goes beyond individuals to the haemophilia community and to keeping it strong. It encompasses the health system and fellow citizens without haemophilia—in terms of both preserving their access to health care, despite the high costs of haemophilia to the budget, and of demonstrating that lives with a health condition are well worth living and there is value in diversity. These cares provide a broad context for choice about even intimate matters like having a baby. Despite an increasing emphasis on self-responsibility in health, members of the haemophilia community also retain a strong sense of citizenship and collective responsibility for managing their condition and moderating costs.

People with haemophilia partake in a changing economy of hope and fear, part of technological networks. Whereas fears used to be about death and serious injury, then about getting effective treatment, and, not too long after, about not getting fatal or debilitating viruses, nowadays, although a trace of those fears persists, with commercially produced products and an overworked health system, the new worry is about continuity of supply and cost. Hope has perhaps not changed as much: more effective, safe, convenient treatment and, with somewhat more scepticism, the elimination of haemophilia altogether.

A particular feature of haemophilia, which is shared with several other genetic conditions, is that of differentiated time. There is the need for urgent, expert treatment in emergencies, best served by a network of care that avoids general Accident and Emergency departments of hospitals and leads straight to the haematology ward or haemophilia treatment centre. But there is also the long view. Most families have had generations of experience with this condition and any new treatment has to stand up to the test of: 'how will this affect future generations', not the usual, relatively short, period of a clinical trial. This deep experience, along with changes in medical professionals' ways of working with one another and with patients, has produced a network of care in which patients (or parents), nurses, physiotherapists and others are also experts, alongside medical specialists, and patients are quite capable of 'doctoring' treatment plans to suit their activities and needs and even changing the national management of their treatment services, as the next chapters detail.

Notes

1. No information from mother or daughter was divulged to the other.
2. In New Zealand, this is 16 years, or earlier if they pass the legal test of Gillick competence, in which the child must be 'of sufficient intellect and maturity to understand fully the nature of what is being proposed' (Ministry of Health 1998; Shenfield 2002, 270).

3. Both CVS and amniocentesis carry an appreciable risk of harm to the foetus or miscarriage. The rate differs from centre to centre but an average is 1 per cent.
4. It is quite common that when people receive the result that their baby does not have a particular condition, they assume the baby is healthy (Buchbinder and Timmerman 2011).

References

Arnold, E., N. Heddle, S. Lane, J. Sek, T. Almonte, and I. Walker. 2005. 'Handheld Computers and Paper Diaries for Documenting the Use of Factor Concentrates Used in Haemophilia Home Therapy: A Qualitative Study'. *Haemophilia* 11 (3):216–26.

Baird, D., L. Geering, K. Saville-Smith, L. Thompson, and T. Tuhipa. 1995. 'Whose Genes are They Anyway? Report of the HRC Conference on Human Genetic Information'. Auckland: Health Research Council.

Brodwin, P. 2000. 'Introduction'. In *Biotechnology and Culture: Bodies, Anxieties, Ethics*, edited by P. Brodwin, 1–26. Bloomington: Indiana University Press.

Buchbinder, M., and S. Timmermans. 2011. 'Medical Technologies and the Dream of the Perfect Newborn'. *Medical Anthropology* 30 (1):56–80.

Cameron, J. 1990. *Why Have Children? A New Zealand Case Study*. Christchurch: University of Canterbury Press.

Canadian Hemophilia Society. 2018. 'History of Hemophilia'. https://www. hemophilia.ca/history-of-hemophilia/ (last accessed 11 Nov, 2018).

Carnahan, M. 2003. 'Towards a Partnership of Care for Patients with Haemophilia'. *New Zealand Medical Journal* 116 (1187):721–22.

Coopers and Lybrand. 1995. *Prophylactic Treatment for Severe Haemophilia A: An Assessment of Costs and Benefits*. Wellington: Ministry of Health. http://www.moh. govt.nz/notebook/nbbooks.nsf/0/38ECC3AA544C56784C256849007FC363? OpenDocument (last accessed 11 Nov, 2018).

Cowan, R.S. 1994. 'Women's Roles in the History of Amniocentesis and Chorionic Villi Sampling'. In *Women and Prenatal Testing: Facing the Challenges of Genetic Technology*, edited by K.H. Rothenberg and E.J. Thomson, 35–48. Columbus: Ohio State University Press.

Dixon, J.W., I. Winship, and D.R. Webster. 1995. 'Priorities for Genetic Services in New Zealand'. A Report to the National Advisory Committee on Core Health and Disability Support Services.

Faed, J. 2003. 'Haemophilia Treatment: Where to from Here? Have the Risks Increased?'. *New Zealand Medical Journal* 116 (1180):559–61.

Forman, J., and O. Baddeley. 2013. *Pre-implantation Genetic Diagnosis: Seven Years' Experience in New Zealand*. Wellington: New Zealand Organisation for Rare Disorders (NZORD).

Gates, E.A. 1994. 'Does Testing Benefit Women?'. In *Women and Prenatal Testing: Facing the Challenges of Genetic Technology*, edited by K.H. Rothenberg and E.J. Thomson, 183–200. Columbus: Ohio State University Press.

Govern, J., and J. Wuthnow. 2004. 'Challenging Scientific Legitimacy: Citizen Participation and Technoscience'. In *Challenging Science: Issues for New Zealand Society in the 21st Century*, edited by K. Dew and R. Fitzgerald, 51–67. Palmerston North: Dunmore Books.

Franklin, S., and C. Roberts. 2006. *Born and Made: An Ethnography of Pre-Implantation Genetic Diagnosis*. Princeton: Princeton University Press.

Harper, P., M. Brasser, L. Moore, L. Teague, L. Pitcher, and P. Ockelford. 2003. 'The Challenge Arising from the Cost of Haemophilia Care: An Audit of Treatment at Auckland Hospital'. *New Zealand Medical Journal* 115 (1180):561–70.

Heath, D., R. Rapp, and K-S. Taussig. 2007. 'Genetic Citizenship'. In *A Companion to the Anthropology of Politics*, edited by D. Nugent and J. Vincent, 152–57. Malden MA: Blackwell Publishing.

High, K.A., and M.W. Skinner. 2011. 'Editorial: Cell Phones and Landlines: The Impact of Gene Therapy on the Cost and Availability of Treatment for Hemophilia'. *Molecular Therapy* 19 (10):1749–50.

Hogben, S., and P. Boddington. 2006. 'The Rhetorical Construction of Ethical Positions: Policy Recommendations for Non-Therapeutic Genetic Testing in Childhood'. *Communication & Medicine* 3 (2):135–46.

IHC. 1995. 'Prenatal Testing'. *Community Moves* 33(2).

Jutel, A.G. 2011. *Putting a Name to it: Diagnosis in Contemporary Society*. Baltimore: Johns Hopkins University Press.

Latour, B. 1987. *Science in Action: How to Follow Scientists and Engineers Through Society*. Cambridge: Harvard University Press.

———. 2002. 'Morality and Technology: The End of the Means'. Translated by Couze Venn. *Theory, Culture & Society* 19 (5/6): 247–60.

Ljung, R., S. Kling, and U. Tedgård. 1995. 'The Impact of Prenatal Diagnosis on the Incidence of Haemophilia in Sweden'. *Haemophilia* 1:190–3.

Ministry of Health. 1998. *Consent in Child and Youth Health*. Wellington: MOH.

Mol, A. 2002. *The Body Multiple: Ontology in Medical Practice*. Durham: Duke University Press.

———. 2008. *The Logic of Care: Health and the Problem of Patient Choice*. Abingdon, Oxon, and New York: Routledge.

National Advisory Committee on Health and Disability. 2003. 'Molecular Genetic Testing in New Zealand'. Wellington: National Health Committee.

[NBTSAC] National Blood Transfusion Services Advisory Committee. 1994. 'Haemophilia: The Supply and Usage of Factor VIII'. Auckland: NBTSAC.

National Hemophilia Foundation [US]. 2018a. 'History of Bleeding Disorders'. https://www.hemophilia.org/Bleeding-Disorders/History-of-Bleeding-Disorders (last accessed 11 Nov, 2018).

———. 2018b. 'Steps for Living'. https://stepsforliving.hemophilia.org/basics-of-bleeding-disorders/genetics-of-bleeding-disorders/hemophilia-carrier-testing# whoshouldbetested (last accessed 11 Nov, 2018).

NIH National Institutes of Health. 2014. 'Gene Therapy—A Revolution in Progress'. https://history.nih.gov/exhibits/genetics/sect4.htm (last accessed 11 Nov, 2018).

Novas, C. 2006. 'The Political Economy of Hope: Patients' Organizations, Science and Biovalue'. *Biosocieties* (3):289–305.

Oliver, M. 1990. *The Politics of Disablement*. London: Macmillan.

Park, J. 1998. 'Technologies for Prenatal Testing: Consequences for Women and Families with an Inherited Condition'. *Pacific Science Association Information Bulletin* 49 (3–4):33–37.

———. 2000. '"The Only Hassle is You Can't Play Rugby": Haemophilia and Masculinity in New Zealand'. *Current Anthropology* 41:443–52.

———. 2005. 'Beyond "His Sisters and His Cousins and His Aunts": Discourses of Haemophilia and Women's Experiences in New Zealand'. In *A Polymath*

Anthropologist: Essays in Honour of Ann Chowning, RAL 6, edited by C. Gross, H.D. Lyons, and D.A. Counts, 97–104. Auckland: University of Auckland.
———. 2009. 'Concepts of Human Nature, Personhood and Natural-Normal in New Reproductive Technology Discourses in New Zealand'. *Anthropologica* 51:173–186.
———. 2013. 'Painful exclusion: Hepatitis C in the New Zealand Haemophilia Community'. In *Senses and Citizenships: Embodying Political Life,* edited by S. Trnka, C. Dureau, and J. Park, 221–41. New York: Routledge.
Park, J., and R. Fitzgerald. 2011. 'Biotechnologies of Care'. In *A Companion to Medical Anthropology,* edited by M. Singer and P.A. Erickson, 425–42. New York: Wiley Blackwell.
Park, J., and B. Strookappe. 1996. 'Deciding About Having Children in Families with Haemophilia'. *New Zealand Journal of Disability Studies* 3:51–67.
Park, J., and D. York. 2008. *The Social Ecology of New Technologies and Haemophilia in New Zealand: 'A Bleeding Nuisance' Revisited.* RAL 8.Department of Anthropology, The University of Auckland. https://researchspace.auckland.ac.nz/handle/2292/4534 (last accessed 11 Nov, 2018).
Pruthi, R.K. 2005. 'Hemophilia: A Practical Approach to Genetic Testing'. *Mayo Clinic Proceedings* 80 (11):1485–99.
Rabinow, P., and N. Rose. 2006. 'Biopower Today'. *BioSocieties* 1 (2):195–211.
Rapp, R. 1991. 'Moral Pioneers: Women, Men and Foetuses on a Frontier of Reproductive Technology'. In *Gender at the Cross-Roads of Knowledge,* edited by M. di Leonardo, 383–95. Berkeley: University of California Press.
———. 1993. 'Accounting for Amniocentesis'. In *Knowledge, Power and Practice: The Anthropology of Medicine and Everyday Life,* edited by S. Lindenbaum and M. Lock, 55–76. Berkeley: University of California Press.
Rose, N. 2006. *The Politics of Life Itself: Biomedicine, Power, and Subjectivity in the Twenty-First Century.* Princeton, NJ: Princeton University Press.
Ross, J. 1997. 'The Perspectives of Haemophilia Carriers'. *World Federation of Hemophilia Pacific Rim Workshop Papers* 8:1–7.
Rothman, B.K. 1994. 'The Tentative Pregnancy: Then and Now'. In *Women and Prenatal Testing: Facing the Challenges of Genetic Technology,* edited by K.H. Rothenberg and E.J. Thomson, 260–70. Columbus: Ohio State University Press.
Scott, A., and B. Tipene-Matua. 2004. 'Cultural Conflict and New Biotechnologies. What is at Risk?'. In *Challenging Science: Issues for New Zealand Society in the 21st century.* In K. Dew, and R. Fitzgerald, 126–45. Palmerston North: Dunmore Books.
Shakespeare, T. 2006. *Disability Rights and Wrongs.* London: Routledge.
Shenfield, F. 2002. 'Ethical Issues in the Genetic Aspects of Haemophilia'. *Haemophilia,* 8:268–72.
Taylor, J.S. 2000. 'Of Sonograms and Baby Prams: Prenatal Diagnosis, Pregnancy, and Consumption'. *Feminist Studies* 26 (2):391–418.
Tedgård, U. 1998. 'Carrier Testing and Prenatal Diagnosis of Haemophilia-Utilisation and Psychological Consequences'. *Haemophilia* 4:365–9.
Titmuss, R. 1970. *The Gift Relationship: From Human Blood to Social Policy.* London: Allen and Unwin.
Trnka, S. 2017. *One Blue Child: Asthma, Responsibility, and the Politics of Global Health.* Stanford, CA: Stanford University Press.

Van de Water, N.S., P.A. Ockelford, E.W. Berry, and P.J. Browett. 1991. 'Haemophilia Management: The Application of DNA Analysis for Prenatal Diagnosis'. *New Zealand Medical Journal* 104:443–46.

Wane, J. 2004. 'Blood Ties: Heartbreak Over Choice for Abortion'. *Sunday Star Times*, January 25.

Weinstein, M.C., G. Torrance, and A. McGuire 2009. 'QALYs: The Basics'. *Value in Health* 12 Supplement 1:S5–S9.

Williams, C., J. Sandall, G. Lewando-Hundt, B. Heyman, K. Spencer, and R. Grellier, 2005. 'Women as Moral Pioneers? Experiences of First Trimester Antenatal Screening'. *Social Science and Medicine* 61 (9):1983–92.

World Federation of Hemophilia. 2014. 'The Clotting Process'. https://www.wfh.org/en/page.aspx?pid=635 (last accessed 11 Nov, 2018).

———. 2015. 'History of the WFH'. https://www.wfh.org/en/about-us/50-years-of-advancing-treatment-for-all (last accessed 11 Nov, 2018).

Zola, I.K. 1977. 'Aging and Disability: Toward a Unifying Agenda'. In *Growing Old in America*, edited by D.H. Fischer, 219–39. New York: Oxford University Press.

5 The shadow on our lives
Hepatitis C in the haemophilia community

Justin and hepatitis C: an introduction

Justin, a young married man when Deon interviewed him in 2006, learned that he had hepatitis C shortly after he started high school. He and his brother had moderate haemophilia so were treated infrequently at home with clotting factor. Nonetheless, both became infected. For Justin, it was 'the worst thing' about having haemophilia and 'the shadow on your life' that meant he 'did not know what [his] life expectancy was'. His goal through high school was to live to age 26: a goal achieved.

Like many others, Justin and his brother found out their hepatitis C status in 1992. They were told by their doctor that no one knew much about hepatitis C, and it was possible they could live their whole lives without it affecting them, but some people did get sick with it. Justin explained that no one really talked about hepatitis C at home, the idea being that if it did start to affect them, they would talk about it then. He almost forgot about it, except it was 'always there at the back of my mind', and it did sometimes come up, such as with close friends or during his visits to the haemophilia centre.

About 2000 or 2002, he recalled, he was contacted by his haemophilia centre and a staff member suggested he visit a gastroenterologist. He had left home at this point and decided that he wanted to take ownership of this illness and find out what was going on, as he did not know much about it. For example, he had a period of depression that he said was because he thought he could not have children (because of the virus) and he really wanted children. A big break-through in terms of finding credible information and a network of people with similar problems occurred for him at a hepatitis C conference in Wellington early in 2005. He was not involved much with the haemophilia community until then, and he found it very reassuring to meet so many people who shared his experiences.

In 2005, he started the (then) new treatment regimen of pegylated interferon and ribavirin for up to 12 months and was still on it during his interview. Subsequently, he became hepatitis C-free. Deon asked him about his experiences with the treatment, and specifically asked about side-effects, something that typically Justin tried to ignore himself and did not talk about to others. He revealed that he felt tired, had flu symptoms the whole time, burned easily in the sun, overheated easily, lacked energy, lost his appetite, and lost a lot of weight: the embodiment of three year's work in the gym on building up muscle. He had periods of being very short-tempered, suffered depression, and had skin problems such as rashes and athlete's foot.

When he began his treatment, he had recently finished his university degree and had just started a new job. Although he was anxious about his lowered capacity for work, his boss was very understanding and encouraging. Reflecting on how he felt during his treatment, Justin said, despite the symptoms listed above, 'from what they've said it could be and how it has been, I've been really, really lucky'. Later he added, 'As long as I can walk and stuff, I'm pretty happy, eh? I just look at that and say, "Well at least I can walk!" ' (Park and York 2008, 46).

Justin's story encapsulates the experiences and values of many of the men, and the few women, who contracted hepatitis C through clotting factor replacement, and shows common themes of uncertainty, pervasiveness, and stoicism. Although Justin did not pay it too much attention, the shadow of hepatitis C was always there in the background. His family coped by putting off discussion until there was an acute need, but at a certain point, he took control, became a self-managing, active patient, learned much more about it and became part of a network of informed and supportive people with haemophilia and hepatitis C. However, the uncertainty of the progress of the disease, and the quality and outcome of treatment was still there. Justin thought carefully about when to have the treatment, waiting until he was in good employment with an understanding employer. Despite the very serious side effects that he incurred, he cleared the virus and felt 'lucky' in view of other possible outcomes of this disease. His simple hope: 'as long as I can walk', reminds us that as a young man with haemophilia, were it not for the blood products that gave him the hepatitis C, he might not be walking unaided. The story is redolent of stoicism: both his and his family's.

Our goal in this chapter is to examine personal and community suffering incurred by people with haemophilia as a result of contracting viruses, especially hepatitis C, through their health service-provided haemophilia treatment. We show that the social context, including diverse understandings of the viruses, state funded health services, and accident compensation arrangements, became an integral part of the experience of hepatitis C for people with haemophilia and the wider haemophilia community: the political is personal, and embodied. The experience of hepatitis C, in turn, was shaped by the then recent and continuing tragedy of HIV. We interpret the local biology of haemophilia and hepatitis C in New Zealand through the concept of social suffering.

Social suffering is about what various forms of power do to people (Kleinman, Das, and Lock 1997, ix). In this case, the local biology of haemophilia and hepatitis C involves a genetic condition that impedes blood clotting and a destructive bioform, hepatitis C, which is a virus that damages the liver and can make a person feel wretched. It also includes community institutions that may support, stigmatise, or ignore these conditions, and the State that controls the health services and access to compensation for harms suffered. Through its policies and agents, the State acts in very intimate ways with people with haemophilia. We argue that part of the suffering with haemophilia and hepatitis C has 'its origins and consequences in the devastating injuries that social force can inflict on human experience' (Kleinman, Das, and Lock 1997, ix), casting, as Justin explained, 'a shadow on our lives'. The most pertinent social force was exerted by the Department (later Ministry) of Health and ACC.

The story begins with a brief review of HIV in the haemophilia community before moving to a detailed discussion of living under the shadow of hepatitis C. We show how our developing understanding of hepatitis C as our research unfolded paralleled scientific development of knowledge about and treatment of hepatitis C, the growing realisation within the haemophilia community that treatment products were contaminated by hepatitis C and that this may have serious consequences for their health and life. We conclude the chapter with a comparison of the experiences of New Zealanders with haemophilia and hepatitis C in relation to the citizens of some comparable countries. This leads into our analysis of organisational interactions, and politics and a detailed analysis of the social forces involved, the subject of chapter 6.

HIV

Ten years before our research began, people living with haemophilia in New Zealand learned that HIV had been detected in the blood supply. This came just one month after health authorities reported they were confident that 'haemophiliacs' in New Zealand were not at risk from AIDS. In November 1984, the headline that the community had been dreading, 'Blood tainted by AIDS', appeared in the *Auckland Star* newspaper (1984). Clinicians had warned of the risk to the blood supply almost a year earlier (Berry and Wyld 1983). Through the media, the Blood Service revealed that a factor IX product, prothrombinex, used in New Zealand, had been manufactured from plasma that may have had AIDS antibodies. This product—Batch 694—had been distributed and used from August 1984. It transpired that the recently privatised CSL Bioplasma had been topping-up New Zealand with Australian blood. However, as the first diagnosis of AIDS in New Zealand was made in 1984 (Dickson and Paul 1996), even separating New Zealand from Australian blood may not by itself have protected the blood supply, though it is possible it might have delayed contamination.

The Minister of Health, with prompting by the Haemophilia Society and its Medical Advisory Committee, moved quickly to authorise safety measures: stricter donor screening, expansion of testing programmes, upskilling laboratory workers, withdrawal of the affected products and viral inactivation. From early in 1985, there has been no HIV infection through the blood supply. In Auckland, attempts were made to produce both factor VIII and IX, and the Department of Health recommended the use of cryoprecipitate from selected donors, which was applicable to haemophilia A only. As a result of the shortage of products for people with haemophilia A, the lack of products for haemophilia B, and the fears about safety, many people at this time were inadequately treated for their bleeding problems, and suffer joint damage and other ill effects to this day. In all, 28 people with haemophilia were infected with HIV through the New Zealand blood supply and one New Zealander was believed to have been infected overseas.

This suffering shaped a shared sense of grief and fear for their futures in this small interconnected haemophilia community; two emotions that were particularly evident during our research in the mid-1990s. By this time, 11 of the 28 people infected by HIV had died. We interviewed 13 people with HIV, some of whom had also contracted hepatitis C. Several have since died. These people are sorely missed and keenly remembered by individuals, families, friends, researchers, and the whole community. The NZHS developed remembrance ceremonies for those who died of AIDS, now including all who have died. The national newsletter, *Bloodline,* also carries obituaries for those who have passed away.

Some of the people who were infected with HIV were young children. One of them was a young dare devil. At haemophilia camps, everyone held their breath as he took part in what seemed like scary activities for such a frail little person, such as zooming down an enormous water slide at breakneck speed. He was taken into the heart of the community and we could see a common thought written on people's faces as their attention was riveted on him flying through the air: 'But why not. He should live life to the full as he is going to have so little of it'. Some community members found the process of coming to the annual haemophilia camps or other get-togethers and seeing how the boys and men deteriorated with AIDS, in this period before effective treatment, too hard to bear. The new generation antiretrovirals came too late for most and a cohort is missing.

The entire haemophilia community had become the object of public scrutiny because of the HIV epidemic. Fear and discrimination were rife (see Box 5.1). The Haemophilia Society challenged the media, particularly the former *Auckland Star,* for their barrage of articles that exacerbated public fears about HIV and AIDS. Suspicion and ignorance about HIV served to stigmatise the whole haemophilia population and forced those who had contracted the virus to grapple with disclosure issues, not just about HIV but about haemophilia, so close was the association in public consciousness.

What happened, more particularly with HIV but also with hepatitis C; haemophiliacs got this thing [HIV] and then family by family they shrivelled up into little balls and dealt with it the best way they could and there

---

Box 5.1

Headlines relating to AIDS

Some headlines demonstrate the depth of public fear such as 'Prosecute Those Giving Blood Knowing They Have AIDS', *'Ban Male Donors'*, *'AIDS Fear has Some Seeking Own Donors'*, *'AIDS Fear Prompts Appeal to Dr Bassett'*.

Others seemed to be designed to stimulate public concern—*'AIDS Epidemic on the Way'*, *'Dentists Cover Up'*, *'AIDS Virus Carriers Found in NZ'*, *'Rugby Kids at Risk of AIDS'*, *'Transfusion Induced AIDS Inevitable'* *'Bedbugs Linked to AIDS Spread'*.

Still others show the concerns of particular occupational groups—*'AIDS Flight Angers* [Air] *Crew'*, *'Police Fears of Contact With Saliva'*.

Others were just generally alarming—*'AIDS Will Strike Thousands in New Zealand'* and *'AIDS Time Bomb'*.

---

was nobody that took up the banner and fought for them. It was too much of a great tragedy.

(Member of the haemophilia community)

As this man suggests, HIV was such a devastating blow that some families coped by turning inward in their sorrow. However, as chapter 6 demonstrates, there was a collective response. NZHS was there to support those who were able to acknowledge that a family member had HIV, and later hepatitis C. It was able to help families and individuals on a very personal level through the care offered by volunteers and the work of an outreach worker, and to help fight for their rights in the community and with the State. The Society advocated for people with HIV who were being excluded from school, employment or other daily activities. A two-month battle to have a Canterbury boy with haemophilia treatment-acquired HIV accepted at a local school is one example of many (Carnahan 2013, 18).

Yet even in this situation, some participants found they were able to value the life that had been afforded them by blood products, while angry and uncertain of their futures with HIV:

...the blood products, although they will bring around my ultimate death, they have given me the opportunity to live. If it wasn't for the blood products I'd be crippled up in a hospital bed somewhere.

(Young man with HIV who was well enough to pursue his profession in 1995, but died in the subsequent decade)

It was in the shadow of the experience of HIV that members of the haemophilia community were confronted by and confronted hepatitis C.

The idea that a similar tragedy could unfold was almost unbearable. And with a much higher proportion of people with haemophilia infected with hepatitis C than had been infected with HIV, their fears of renewed discrimination were very acute.

Learning together about hepatitis C

Before we began our research, we were well aware of the traumas of HIV and AIDS for people with haemophilia, but the great importance of hepatitis C was only revealed to us when we began our pilot studies to finalise our research design and methods. We were advised by NZHS committee members and other people with haemophilia to include questions about hepatitis C and about accident compensation in our postal questionnaire and focus groups. In view of the results from these questions we included discussions about hepatitis C in our interviews in 1994–5 and in each of the subsequent studies, and attended workshops and conferences about hepatitis C. We sought to understand and describe the physical and social effects of hepatitis C, and of the treatment for hepatitis C for people with haemophilia in New Zealand. We wanted to document the embodied experience of hepatitis C to complement statistical accounts of the epidemic. We learned that people with hepatitis C were not just contending with a virus but with many other challenges. These included uncertainty and confusion about what having the virus meant, lack of validation of their disease by health professionals and others, poor health services, and discrimination. It was all these together that constituted the local biology of haemophilia and hepatitis C.

As we proceeded with our initial study, we found that the realisation of the importance of hepatitis C was spreading through the haemophilia community, but some people were only just becoming familiar with it. One man, for example, very cheerfully told us that he had antibodies to hepatitis C. When we enquired further, not being able to understand why he seemed pleased about his antibodies, we discovered that he thought it meant that he was now immune to it, rather than that he had been exposed to it and might have developed chronic infection.

In 1994–5, 12 per cent of our 193 participants were unaware of their hepatitis C status, and 84 had been diagnosed positive. Ten of those with hepatitis C also had HIV or AIDS. We routinely advised those who did not know their status to contact their health professionals or haemophilia outreach worker and we gave out written information supplied by the hepatitis C support group and the NZHS on request. It was not until 2003 that HFNZ was able to establish with some confidence the number of people in their community who had been infected with hepatitis C. Their comprehensive 2003 survey found that 189 people had been infected (Carnahan 2013, 39). Many people had also had hepatitis B one or more times over the years as a result of haemophilia treatment.

It was not surprising that knowledge of 'hep C', as it was usually referred to, was not universal in the haemophilia community. The virus had been identified as an RNA virus only in 1989 and its natural history was not well-understood (Alter and Klein 2008; Choo *et al.* 1989). From the midtwentieth century, serum hepatitis, eventually known as hepatitis B, and another hepatitis, referred to as 'non-A non-B', were known to be present in blood transfusions and, later, present in blood products. Even after hepatitis C had been identified, there was much uncertainty about what hepatitis C did, what its effects were, how to keep it out of the blood supply, and how to treat it.

Although it could not be directly tested for until after it was identified, from 1986 'surrogate testing', i.e., testing for something commonly associated with it, such as hepatitis B, was available, and if used and acted upon, it could have excluded a large proportion of hepatitis C from blood products. Uptake of these less-than-perfect surrogate tests was variable across different health jurisdictions and was not used in New Zealand. Hepatitis C antibodies could also be tested for but, again, accuracy was a problem and there was always a window during which infection might have occurred but no antibodies yet produced. Antibody tests were available from 1988 and were made commercially available in 1990, but not generally used in New Zealand except in a series of sentinel tests reported by the Auckland Blood Bank Director, Dr Graeme Woodfield in 1991 (Woodfield 1991). These tests showed a frequency of hepatitis C of 0.5% in blood donors and a 65% frequency in the 45 people with haemophilia whose blood was tested. Direct tests for hepatitis C RNA became available in 2001 and their accuracy progressively improved over the next year (Carnahan 2013, 27–8). The lack of certainty and disagreement in the medical and scientific communities about the natural history and consequences of this long-existing but 'new' disease, hepatitis C, led to great variation across international health services in the uptake of the different generations of tests.

Difficulties with testing for this virus were paralleled by difficulties in removing it from the blood supply. Eventually, superheat treatment of blood products (80°C for 72 hours) was found to inactivate the virus, and other methods, e.g., solvent detergent inactivation, also had some success (Taylor and Power 2011). A superheated product was available in New Zealand for people with haemophilia A from June 1991, but the equivalent product for haemophilia B was slower to become available and not introduced into New Zealand until February 1993 (Carnahan 2013, 26–7).

In December 1989, the New Zealand Blood Transfusion Advisory Committee (BTAC) obtained funding from the Department of Health to carry out tests to determine what proportion of 'at risk' New Zealanders had contracted hepatitis C. This prelude to full-scale testing was completed by June 1990. It was estimated that 70 per cent of people treated with blood products for their haemophilia had hepatitis C (Department of Health 1992). The BTAC chairperson and the New Zealand Communicable

Disease Control Advisory Committee wrote to the Minister of Health and the Director-General of Health advising that testing of blood for hepatitis C should begin immediately. The Minister referred any decision about the implementation of testing back to the Department of Health (Howden-Chapman 1994). It was a full two years before national testing was implemented and two-and-a-half years before all blood products for haemophilia treatment were virus-free because, unconscionably, some old stock made from untested plasma or plasma that had not been high-heat-treated was used up first, i.e., transfused into patients.

At this time, the natural history of hepatitis C was not well understood, partly because it is often a silent disease with a slow onset and nonspecific symptoms. Many clinicians thought of it as a minor irritant rather than a serious disease. It is now established that around 25 per cent of those who become infected can clear the virus autonomously. About half of the 75 per cent who develop a chronic form of hepatitis C will experience some liver damage, usually after 15 to 20 years. This can range from relatively mild to extensive cirrhosis, liver failure, or liver cancer. A small number of those infected experience debilitating symptoms and diminished quality of life right from the outset, whereas others are symptomless (Chen and Morgan 2006; Ministry of Health 2013). In New Zealand, only acute infections with hepatitis C are notified, so the estimation of 50,000 infected from all sources, living with the virus, is very difficult to confirm as is the natural history of the disease in New Zealand.[1]

In the mid-1990s there was still a dismissive attitude expressed by some medical professionals and health and accident compensation officials in New Zealand about the seriousness of hepatitis C. This provides a good example of diffuse medical power operating along interconnected networks. For example, one of our research group members was Dr Elizabeth Berry, at that time a Consultant Haematologist at Auckland Hospital, and a very respected senior health professional. Yet even she was greeted with scepticism when she presented the hepatitis C findings from our initial study at a medical conference in New Zealand in 1995. The suffering of people with hepatitis C was trivialised by some in her medical audience. 'Compensationitis' was one response to her account of their suffering. Her attempts to describe the everyday experience of people with haemophilia and hepatitis C to this medical audience to secure recognition of their illness, instead provoked claims of patient fraudulence. The discrediting reference was to our participants' attempts to receive ACC compensation. Simultaneously, Dr Berry and our research results were discredited. Our experiences with hepatitis C in these early days of the epidemic paralleled the many ways in which our participants' attempts to be taken seriously had been discredited.

Our participants too, when trying to describe their vague flu-like symptoms and fatigue to their GPs, were sometimes met with dismissive responses like, 'Yes, I get tired too'. The exceptions to these dismissals were a small number of gastroenterologists who worked directly with people with haemophilia. 'Permission to be ill' (Nettleton 2006, 1167) was very frequently withheld by GPs. But tiredness, unlike hepatitis C, does not lead to liver damage and cancer. It has been a relief over the last several years to see hepatitis C taken much more seriously by members of the medical profession, and to learn from more recent participants that they and their GPs are better informed about the infection, its possible consequences, and its treatment. But as Nettleton (2006) discusses, a diagnosis like that of hepatitis C brings both certainty and uncertainty, because the effects and progression of hepatitis C are so variable between individuals. Nonetheless, hepatitis C provides a good example of how slowly, over many years, an illness with vague and often subjective symptoms comes to be constituted as a disease after considerable struggle by persons with it and their specialist health professionals. Until the disease is known and recognised by their doctors, people with it cannot occupy the sick role (Parsons 1951) with its rights and obligations, benefits and limitations.

When our study began, there were few accounts of living with hepatitis C in New Zealand or Australia. Over the years, the number of studies grew although the numbers of participants involved was still quite modest. Comparison of our findings with other studies allowed us to see that the findings were robust. It is important to remember that for people with haemophilia, hepatitis C is an additional health problem, and sometimes it is in addition to other infections, especially HIV and hepatitis B. Through our research, our informal discussions, and formal presentations we became part of the emergent dialogue about the seriousness of the virus and the suffering linked to it.

To complement studies of hepatitis C that only quantified incidence and symptoms, we provided details of people's lived experiences, and, because the symptoms were shared with so many other illnesses, how difficult it was not just to get a diagnosis, but for that diagnosis to be accorded significance— especially in the 1980s when there was no specific test. Uncertainty, unpredictability, vagueness of the symptoms, and the difficulties of deciding whether and when to undertake gruelling treatment, which may or may not eradicate the virus, were all part of this experience. These uncertainties and vagaries of hepatitis C layered upon and intersected with other uncertainties and contingencies of living with haemophilia and with being misunderstood or maligned by more powerful actors in the network of care. We trace the story of how people came to understand that, as one person put it, they were 'in trouble', and how they responded.

Symptoms and their cause: an insidious effect

Fatigue, depression, aches, and pains; generalised symptoms such as these could apply to so many different conditions and are difficult to attribute to any one thing. As is often the case with diagnosis of diffuse sets of chronic symptoms, merely recognising the cause of such symptoms, a diagnosis, can be helpful in learning to cope and in making helpful changes to daily routines.

People learned about their hepatitis C diagnoses in a variety of ways. A mother was grateful for the careful explanation given to her and her young boys when their positive hepatitis C results came back from the lab, yet she was so shocked she could not take the information in. On the way home in the car, one of the boys asked, 'Am I going to die?' A young man was satisfied that his doctor had told him plainly and advised him to 'be careful what [he] did with his blood and his sperm'. But others found out by chance—one by a visitor reading the notes on the end of his friend's hospital bed; another by a phone call from his haemophilia nurse advising him to get his claim in to ACC before the closing date—this was the first he had heard that he had hepatitis C. People who found out in this indirect way were angry at the lack of care and consideration, and sometimes the basic inefficiency of communication, exhibited by their health service providers.

In our 1995 interviews with around 80 people, nearly 60 per cent (23 out of 39) of interviewees who knew they had hepatitis C had experienced no clear symptoms. As one person in the study reflected, 'Hepatitis C seems to affect different people in so many different ways. There's no set pattern of what it is going to do'. Those who had experienced fatigue and other health effects of the virus talked about the profound impact that it had on their lives. A few respondents were aware that damage to their liver had already commenced and they were 'in trouble'. Most, however, had been reassured by their doctors that they 'would be well for a long time yet'.

Fatigue or lethargy were most commonly reported. Other symptoms included headaches, depression, and flu-like symptoms such as body and bone aches. One man commented that 'tiredness has an insidious effect, it creeps up on you so you hardly notice but it has a very pervasive effect on daily life'. One frustration was that tiredness tended to be intermittent and unpredictable. A person might feel extremely tired for a period of two or three days, then feel well for several days or weeks. As one man explained, a builder by trade who had had to give up work due to hepatitis C and other health complications, some days he felt like he would like to 'get into something' but other days he had no energy for work. This caused considerable frustration and feelings of being unable to control his life, something echoed by several other respondents. People with extreme symptoms talked about feeling 'spaced out' at times, describing it variously as 'a fog', 'a cotton cobweb', or 'going on a trip'.

Hepatitis C was also a baffling condition. People reported that there was not always a correlation between liver function tests and the existence of symptoms. For example, one woman reported that one of her sons had high alanine aminotransferase levels, which should indicate liver damage, prior to treatment with interferon, yet experienced no symptoms. However, her other son had normal levels but did have symptoms of hepatitis C. These mismatches between the kind of hepatitis C that was indicated by liver function tests and the kind that was experienced by people with it made it particularly difficult to make decisions about timing of treatment, as Mol (2002) described for diabetes.

Several respondents stated that they were unsure if their intermittent fatigue was due to hepatitis C, but it was so commonly reported by people with hepatitis C (for example, by those attending the 1999 Australasian Conference on hepatitis C)[2] that it is difficult to discount. One specialist, a participant in our research who treated many people with haemophilia, commented that the 'subtleties of symptoms can be very difficult to attribute to anything' and said (in 1999) that he was not aware of anyone having major clinical problems such as liver failure. Nevertheless, fatigue and depression make life more difficult, for the patients and their families, because of the moodiness and fluctuating energy levels of the person with it, along with the ongoing worry for their welfare and concerns about infection control.

In both our later studies, we talked in detail with participants about hepatitis C. By this time, diagnoses were more certain and 15 people in each phase knew that they, or a close family member about whom they spoke, had contracted it. As in our earlier studies, each person's experience was different: some had very debilitating symptoms, some very mild. Several people whom we had met earlier feeling very unwell had cleared the virus through treatment, whereas others had progressed to liver disease and we learned that a small number had died.

The uncertainty and unpredictability that undermined one's sense of control was a key theme also reported by Garret and Conrad (2001) for people with hepatitis C in Queensland. That unpredictability was not confined to symptoms only, but to how other people might respond if they knew a person had hepatitis C. The unpredictability of a chronic stigmatised illness and the uncertainty about how it would affect one on a day-to-day, let alone a long-term basis, were major concerns in Queensland and New Zealand. Gifford (1999) too reported on the loss of a sense of control and hope reported by some of the Australian women she interviewed, due to the prejudice and exclusion they experienced. Some members of the Crossen *et al.* (1999) participant group also reported instances of stigmatisation and worry over being stigmatised. However, this aspect did not seem as marked in this Christchurch study of people who were in touch with a support group. The unpredictability of effects is a finding reported in all but the latter study. That study did, however, stress the great variability of experience among those infected with hepatitis C.

People with haemophilia suffering from the effects of hepatitis C responded in a range of ways, including learning to pace themselves, to get plenty of sleep, and be flexible in what they tried to accomplish in a week, depending on their energy levels. Reducing or eliminating alcohol consumption was a common response to being diagnosed. Several people reported changing their diets, usually by including more fruit and vegetables and avoiding fatty foods. There was general agreement that an improved diet was beneficial as they found fatty foods and alcohol difficult to tolerate. Depression was less commonly reported as a result of hepatitis C, but it was also an effect.

People's responses were intimately linked to their responses to having haemophilia. For example, one man reflected on the kind of up-bringing that boys with haemophilia had and how that prepared them to cope with hepatitis C or HIV.

> ...we were always brought up to be very, very positive and it is almost a head-in-the-sand mentality in a sense, but to survive HIV, hepatitis C, whatever is coming next, we've just got to say 'Oh well, what the heck!', and get on. It has got to be your fundamental attitude to it all. Life is good, I am enjoying myself, I've got a lovely family, I work hard...I am just going to get on...I've been working hard to try and get some sort of recognition for hepatitis C, but nothing I can do will change the past.

To tell or not to tell?

Because hepatitis C is contagious, sufferers face social and ethical dilemmas as well as health consequences. Although hepatitis C is not normally contracted through daily contact and is rarely contracted through sexual contact (1–2 per cent), some people were very concerned about the potential of passing on the virus to loved ones. One of the most fraught issues of having hepatitis C for several men was around commencing intimate relationships. Respondents worried about when and what to tell potential partners about hepatitis C, and feared infecting a partner. For young men in particular, a major issue was fear of disclosing their hepatitis C status and facing possible rejection. When asked about everyday life issues associated with having hepatitis C, one young man responded:

> Having girlfriends, trying to start a relationship. You need to tell them straight away. It is okay with friends and family, they are not concerned about me having it. I had my first relationship and didn't tell her for a while, but I got [really stressed] about it and realised I should have told her straight away. The second relationship, I told her on the first day. She was understanding. You have to tell partners the risks and not lie, better not to wait till the relationship develops to tell.

The stigmatised nature of hepatitis C meant that young people tended to avoid telling their friends about having it. As one young man who could not tolerate alcohol at all explained, fear of disclosing his hepatitis C status meant that it was difficult to justify his abstinence to his mates and to feel part of the social scene, which was alcohol focussed. This nondisclosure of an infection unwittingly contracted during treatment for another condition bothered interviewees, compounding their sense of hurt and shame.

To treat or not to treat?

One of the challenges for people with hepatitis C or their parents was trying to make sense of the information that was available and deciding whether, and when, to seek treatment. A participant in 1995 noted that a period of 20 to 25 years was expected to elapse from first contracting the virus to possible progression on to serious symptoms such as liver disease, and people hoped that they would be part of the group in which liver disease would not develop. As one mother described it, 'it feels like a time clock ticking away but because the boys have both been so well, it may not happen to them'. One person expressed the uncertainty that many people felt: 'It's a numbers game. They can't do a biopsy so just have to rely on statistics. Statistically, 20 per cent go on to chronic, of that 20 per cent a small number go to cirrhosis and some of those get liver cancer'. It was in fact possible, though problematic, to perform a liver biopsy for a person with haemophilia as long as clotting levels were raised to within the normal range first, although any such procedure involved some risk. Occasionally a biopsy was taken while a person with haemophilia was undergoing surgery for something else.

By the 1999 study, most people thought that they had enough information about hepatitis C, but some thought the information was inadequate because it was not personalised into what would happen to them. By then, the statistical probability of progression on to develop cirrhosis was cited as 20 per cent, with 15 per cent of people expected to clear the virus spontaneously, and another 25 per cent to be symptomless (Lee 1999). As one person stated, the problem was finding out which group you might be in.

> I've learned to just keep adjusting the limits of what I can do. Not getting frustrated, because I think frustration is the biggest thing, when you want to do something and you can't do it.

Treatment options and decisions for hepatitis C

Over the years of our research, treatment options for hepatitis C progressed from low to fairly high levels of efficacy in clearing the virus, with debates about the optimum length of treatment. Efficacy depends, among other things, on the strain of the virus one has. Unfortunately, the most pervasive strain in New Zealand proved to be the one that was the most difficult to treat. Other factors in successful treatment were the length of the treatment and the combination of medications as well as the initial viral load. In the 1990s, treatment was funded for only six months, and some felt that this was inadequate. Some were able to pay for a second six months themselves. Funded treatment was increased to 12 months as a 12-month regimen was proven to be more effective. Subsequently, much more effective combinations of drugs have led to many people becoming hepatitis C-free—even those with the hard-to-treat Genotype 1.

A common concern of participants throughout our research was whether to undergo treatment, with the possibility of severe side effects and perhaps no difference in viral status, or to wait for better treatments to become available. When we began our research, it was more common for people to be advised, or decide themselves, to wait and see if and when effects from hepatitis C emerged. A small number did undertake treatment, initially with limited success.

In 1999, a gastroenterologist speaking to the Haemophilia Family Camp, recommended that for best results, the latest research suggested that it was more effective to treat early rather than waiting for serious symptoms to develop. In our 1999 study, seven of the 15 people with hepatitis C had undergone treatment with interferon, and another was part of a clinical trial for combination therapies of interferon with pegylated ribavirin. None of these people had cleared the virus, although three said that the treatment had brought their liver function levels down to more normal levels and that their levels had stayed low.

The high rate of debilitating side effects from treatment for hepatitis C was a major consideration when deciding whether or when to treat. Of the seven people who had undertaken treatment in our 1999 study, five suffered side effects, most commonly flulike symptoms such as lethargy, headaches, general achiness, irritability, and depression. These side effects mirrored the symptoms of hepatitis C, and so it was not surprising that some people were hesitant to treat. Three people suffered depression as a result of treatment, mirroring findings of earlier international research that indicated that 17 per cent of people taking interferon experienced depression and other psychological symptoms (Renault, *et al.* 1987). The person who was undergoing combination therapy explained his approach:

> ... the other thing with hepatitis C, and now with this treatment, that has been important is that I really have to monitor my moods, particularly because treatment has created episodes of depression, and I know they are drug related, but they are very difficult. I have to just remove myself from any situation where I interact with anybody because I know I'm going to be volatile. And I think also not to drive or things like that because I get really cranky then and I just know it is not a good combination really.

In this 1999 study, participants spoke about the tremendous importance of being able to discuss and evaluate treatment options with their doctor in an unhurried and unpressured way. A knowledgeable person to act as a 'sounding board' when deciding about treatment was considered valuable. There was a tendency, though not as frequently reported as in our earlier study, for doctors to discourage treatment if a person was not suffering from serious symptoms of the virus. As one person explained, 'the doctor said, "You won't want treatment, will you?" and that was the attitude'. Our interviewee said that he would rather have had treatment options explained so that he could make an informed choice himself.

Another person had had two sets of treatment for hepatitis C at different time periods and so had first-hand experience of a change in attitudes. While in the most recent treatment period he had received good support and a reasonably sympathetic reception to the difficulty of side effects, during his first treatment he recalled:

> I said to him [clinician] that I was having very bad symptoms, so bad that they had stopped me working, I couldn't concentrate, my memory would just go, and he said 'it is to do with haemophilia, people with haemophilia always wrap themselves up in cotton wool'. I was stunned.

In our 2005–6 study, there was still a lack of clarity about optimum periods of treatment. Some reported that they had cleared the virus with just six months of treatment, others did not clear it even with 12 months. Access to treatment appeared to be much improved, but some people still experienced severe problems with access. One man had been pursuing treatment since 1998 and had contracted hepatitis C well before this:

> I finally got to see a hepatologist who was prepared to do something about it in 2003. At that stage, I was told that because I had hep B and hep C I was not entitled to treatment. My response was, 'Well, surely it's good medicine to at least monitor, you know, what's happening'. And I was told, 'Well, no we don't do that'. We don't have a recall and follow-up system within our clinic, which I expressed amazement at, but, yes, they would arrange another appointment for follow-up, bearing in mind this was April 2003… Got home, and my follow-up appointment arrived and it was for November 2005! Um, their idea of follow-up is not my idea of follow-up … and via my haematologist I asked for a further appointment … So, I saw the hepatologist in February 2005. At that point he said, no, that hep B was no longer an impediment to access, ah, 'We will start treatment immediately' … Bearing in mind that was a February appointment, here we are now into mid-June and I still haven't started treatment … I don't intend to allow the systemic failures of the health system to impact on my liver. (His treatment started before our fieldwork was completed).

This man's experience of difficulties of access was not typical in this study phase, although such experiences were very common in earlier years when criteria for access seemed to keep changing. In 2005, so many people were coming forward for treatment from the growing general population of people with the virus that the gastroenterology services in some DHBs were overwhelmed, including the DHB that this person attended. There were some very long delays in getting the initial specialist appointment. However, once that barrier had been passed, most people started treatment quite promptly.

Finding a good time to have treatment, given that treatment could be debilitating, was very difficult. Some people were hesitant to undergo treatment in case it disrupted their lives too much. One woman waited until her children were old enough to look after themselves, others tried to fit it into study and work commitments. Self-employed people were in a particularly difficult position. Eric, a man in his forties, was contemplating having treatment for his hepatitis C during the time of his interview. He was busy with his business and was inclined to put it off.

> I'm kind of a bit busy to take a year off at the moment .... Hell, I'm dog tired now just because of what I've got to do, let alone any treatment. So, it's not really a good time to do it. So, I'm just waiting for perhaps a better time.

But for this busy man with a family to support there was never going to be a good time.

Interferon treatment undoubtedly is difficult for the patient and it can also be hard for those around him or her. A mother, whose son had had a successful 12-month course of interferon monotherapy when he was a teenager, talked about the difficulties the treatment had caused:

> The first couple of weeks were really grotty. It was really difficult for me to know what of his behaviour was interferon-related or what of his behaviour was ... snotty teenage behaviour that you would not accept. So, I didn't know whether to jump on it and say, 'Hey, this is not OK in our house, you won't speak to me like that, you won't behave like that', or whether just to tolerate it for it's only for the year and, you know what I mean? It was a really difficult year. And I wouldn't actually recommend to anyone else that they do it at that age. But then (voice brightens), because of his youth, and hadn't had the virus for long, actually was in his favour. So yeah, it was a very hard year, but I'm pleased it paid off.

Another mother whose children were born late enough (i.e., after 1992) to be protected from hepatitis C, observed the effects of treatment on her friend's son, who was a few years older than her own:

> I saw him at his worst, I saw him so cut up, so bloody sick from taking his interferon that you actually wondered what was in it for him at the end of it all. It was needles after needles, interferon after interferon, he was sick, sick, sick. He'd gone from a very healthy boy to as sick as a dog the next day. And I guess, years later we can reflect on that and say 'He was bloody lucky' because he had a year's supply of interferon,

that his parents paid the other six months for, because the government would only pay for six months. So, he was lucky because they were told that if he had a 12 months' supply, he would have a better success, survival rate, so that's what they did. And look at him now, one fine healthy young adult.

Having adequate support during treatment was an important consideration. One man voiced his uncertainty about undertaking treatment, since he had to consider, amongst other complicating factors, whether his newly single status would mean that he did not have enough support. Interferon treatment is also stressful for partners, and, as the outreach workers confirmed, they can need a lot of support, to help them through the months of coping with and trying to support a tired, grumpy, depressed, and irritable partner especially if the patient also perceives the partner as a source of irritation. Some sisters also described the pain and fear that their brother's reactions to treatment had caused them: losing many kilos of weight or being too sick to get out of bed for your own birthday.

Hepatitis C and social suffering

The suffering incurred by people with haemophilia in these viral epidemics was a complex mixture of feeling unwell or being very ill, being in pain, living with uncertainty and grief, discrimination and silencing, and, as we now discuss, painful relations with the State. One young man with haemophilia and HIV said in 1994:

> … what I'm really angry about is there's never been any great steaming, huge court case against the Crown where everything would have been examined and would have been aired. And in the end, if somebody was responsible or not isn't necessarily the point either, but it would have been examined and we would have known how this had happened. I mean, you have a small group of New Zealanders who intimately rely on the State for their health care. You can't get blood anywhere else and it's an intimate reliance. If you don't have the blood, you will die.

This man wanted the opportunity to bear witness. This situation contrasted starkly with Ireland, where more than 100 people with haemophilia had contracted HIV from their treatment, and people with haemophilia and their families were able to provide written evidence and speak of their experiences, loss, and grief in front of the Lindsay Tribunal to an attentive public (Government of Ireland 2002). The media published daily bulletins (Daly and Cunningham 2003). In the United States, public submissions on HIV and haemophilia were received by the Institute of Medicine (Resnik 1999). Keshavjee, Weiser, and Kleinman (2001, 1090), who analysed the submissions, described them as an expression of deep memory that 'expresses an enduring experience of extreme suffering which cannot be assuaged or easily transformed back to ordinary life conditions'. Yet in New Zealand, the independent 'Bad Blood' enquiry, which reported in December 1992, provided no such opportunity for people to speak of their pain. Additionally, the terms of reference, which focussed the enquiry after 1 July 1992, excluded most people with haemophilia as nearly all but newly treated people would have been infected before this time (Department of Health 1992). One senior politician, Rt Hon Jenny Shipley, could even be understood as shrugging off responsibility by saying that these people with haemophilia chose to have this treatment knowing that there might be problems. Shipley said in 1992, '75 per cent of haemophiliacs actually had hepatitis C prior to 1990 … they have always known …with consent, that they were exposed to a number of risks' (Shipley 1992), conveniently ignoring that people's lives are dependent on treatment products, or 'If you don't have the blood, you die'. Shipley's statement is a clear example of health constructed as a market commodity, and of fellow citizens as consumers. But in the case of health care, patients cannot know all they need to know to be informed consumers and they cannot return a faulty product. Around the same time, a health official explained that New Zealand did not have to be as careful about blood safety as did Australia because ACC would compensate infected people and thus the Health Department did not have to be concerned about legal liability (TVNZ 1992). In this case, patients were constructed as possible plaintiffs, not as citizens to whom a duty of care should be extended. Many in the haemophilia community experienced these statements as a denial of their citizenship rights and the State's refusal of its duty of care. But individuals' responses were not just political and analytical: they were embodied emotional responses of grief and rage at this lack of care.

Kleinman, Das, and Lock (1997, xiii) suggest that an important question to ask is how social 'suffering is produced in societies and how acknowledgement of pain, as a cultural process, is given or withheld'. The withholding of care evinced by elected representatives of the people and public servants alike contributed to the pain and suffering of people with haemophilia and HIV or hepatitis C. The bureaucratic technical responses to the tragedy suppressed the moral dimension of the issue: that which is symbolised by the desire for acknowledgement of their full citizenship and the harm done (see Figure 5.1).

The sense of not being considered a full citizen worthy of care was very apparent in the descriptions families with haemophilia gave of their experiences in dealing with various arms of the state (Park 2013). Here we mention just a few examples. A mother of two boys with haemophilia who both had been infected with hepatitis C described her 'fight with ACC'. She felt that they had been very badly treated and furthermore that the 'Ministry of Health have never admitted neglect'. Her boys were so mortified about contracting hepatitis C that they were unwilling to speak out about their

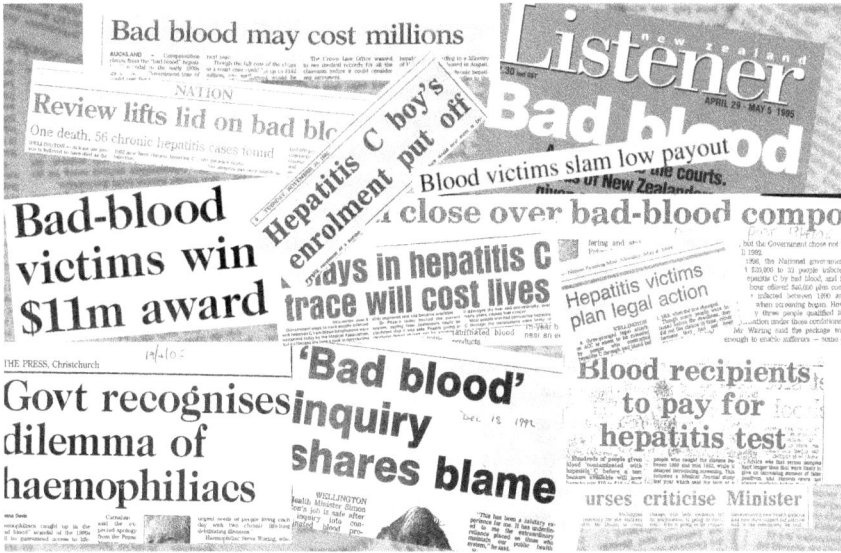

Figure 5.1 Headlines relating to hepatitis C in the blood supply.

unfair treatment, as that would disclose their status. Even the Crown Law Office, which another interviewee had always thought was above politics, was experienced as 'stonewalling people with haemophilia on the hepatitis C issue'. Another participant expressed the view that the delays were in the hope that transfusion-related hepatitis C would die out, to prevent a payout: he implied, of course, that the government was waiting until all the people with transfusion-related hepatitis C died.

Some felt abandoned by the state: Feeling that they were being 'thrown on the rubbish heap' and 'not worth the effort to protect' was how they interpreted, first, the lack of recognition that hepatitis C was causing mental, physical, and social anguish to people with haemophilia, their families, and doctors and, second, after recognition that there was a problem, the glacial speed at which interventions were made. This sense of being treated as if they were worthless was exacerbated by hepatitis C being identified on the heels of HIV. History was repeating itself as a tragedy of neglect. The collective representations and sensitivities created by the haemophilia community's experience with HIV shaped that of hepatitis C.

Working through the HFNZ archives for the late 1980s and 1990s, we read heart-wrenching and angry letters from haematologists entreating the successive Ministers of Health to enact and fund measures such as screening of donors, testing of donations, and high-heat treatment of blood products, to protect their patients from a contaminated blood supply. Letters from NZHS reiterate the same pleas (Carnahan 2013). Meanwhile, to keep people with haemophilia functioning, their doctors had no alternative but to use products that, depending on their batch number, might be, or definitely were, unsafe. Doctors graphically described the dilemma that they were in. One, for example, recalled how he had put a batch of clotting factor on a high shelf. He thought it was almost certainly contaminated. To his relief he managed to get through the period before the safe factor arrived without having to use it. Taylor and Power (2011) describe the same fears and dilemma from Ireland.

Parents were placed in exactly the same position, and described their anguish in infusing their children with products that might infect them, or unwittingly infusing them, and finding out later their child had been infected by a product they themselves had administered, as did this mother with whom we were speaking in 1994, whose son contracted hepatitis C.

> I had a lot of grief with it because I was giving him his treatment and I thought (draws in breath), 'My God, I've done that. I've given him this—even though it's not my blood'.

Some discontinued treatment with blood products, preferring the risk of damaged joints and painful bleeds to hepatitis and its complications. Despite these precautions, some ended up with both damaged joints and hepatitis having unknowingly been infected earlier. When people with haemophilia discovered that unsafe stock had been used up in the interests of economy even after safe products were available, they felt that their lives were judged worthless. This was reinforced some years later when it was discovered that prisoners—a group known to have very high rates of blood-borne viruses—were giving blood long after this practice was supposed to have been stopped (Lauzon 2008, 108).

The collective response from the haemophilia community in New Zealand involved establishment of further outreach workers to help provide extra care for those with hepatitis C and an attempt to engage with the government about redress, ongoing welfare and care, and the future safety of blood products; a response we discuss in chapter 6. The Haemophilia Foundation of New Zealand and individual members experienced tremendous delays in their dealings with the several faces of government, such as the Ministry of Health and the ACC.

ACC as a branch of the State

Part of the local biology of haemophilia and hepatitis C in New Zealand is the network of care in which it is enmeshed. The state institution of ACC is an important node in this network. A great boon for New Zealanders and visitors alike who incur injuries through accidents, ACC's role is more murky in other circumstances that its provisions cover, such as blood-borne viruses contracted through medical means. Additionally, the provisions were not written with chronic diseases of uncertain progression in mind. In

1974, the 1973 ACC Act came into law whereby common law rights were given up in exchange for fair compensation under ACC. ACC covered many of the costs of the treatment of accidents as well as providing to people who qualified up to 80 per cent of their previous income while they recovered or while they were impaired. The 1982 ACC Act allowed all citizens who suffered long-term effects of an accident entitlement to compensation, which was to include those who contracted HIV and hepatitis C through blood or blood products deemed to be 'medical misadventure'. Claimants were entitled to up to $10,000 NZD for pain and suffering plus up to $17,000 NZD for permanent disability or impairment. The 1982 Act was replaced on 1 July 1992 with the Accident and Rehabilitation Compensation Insurance Act 1992, whereupon lump sum payments were abolished, strict time limits for lodging a claim were imposed and definitions of medical misadventure became more restrictive. This was the change that was most consequential for people with haemophilia and hepatitis C.

It is no exaggeration to say that for some, dealing with ACC was an affliction just as surely as was hepatitis C. Changes in the ACC Acts had significant impacts on people's ability to seek redress for hepatitis C and, across time, created huge differences in how people were treated by ACC. By unpacking the meanings and effects of changes to ACC for people with haemophilia, we reveal another important element of social suffering: how people felt abandoned by the state.

Furthermore, differences by region and even by individual ACC officers created further inequities in the response to the chronic and somewhat unpredictable condition of hepatitis C. Claims were processed at the regional level, so there was no group in ACC with expertise in the matter. One hundred of our initial participants had applied for ACC compensation, and three-quarters of those claims had been in relation to hepatitis C. Several of our participants reported that their files and claims had been lost by ACC. Losing files was seen as a strategy rather than simple carelessness by many would-be clients of ACC, especially in the early years. Unhelpfulness and disregard for privacy also characterised the experiences of some would-be claimants.

Although many people in this community would have acquired hepatitis C before the 1990s, they were not eligible for lump-sum compensation because they were unaware that they had the virus when the 1992 Act was introduced and therefore had not submitted their claims in time. Delays in diagnosis and failure of some health professionals to notify patients of the diagnosis of hepatitis C was the reason in many cases, and it was not until the 'bad blood' scandal erupted in the media in November 1992 that many learned that they had hepatitis C, too late for claims to be filed under the old Act.

Under the 1992 Act, claimants were entitled only to an independence allowance, based on the degree of physical disability. The maximum weekly allowance was $40 NZD, although people in our study received between $4 and $20. Some considered it 'too much hassle' for small rewards, and had not bothered to apply, although they were encouraged to do so by the Haemophilia Foundation in case they should require income assistance in the future, should they find themselves unable to work due to hepatitis C.

The concerns of those people interviewed in 1999 in relation to compensation for hepatitis C revolved around the unhelpful treatment they had received from ACC, the inadequate compensation, and the ongoing struggle with the government over the issue. Six of the 15 interviewed had received $10,000 for 'pain and suffering' from ACC, and a further four had received this $10,000 plus a percentage of the $17,000 for permanent disability or impairment (ranging from five to 20 per cent). Four had not received any compensation as they had not made their claims in time and one had received only medical costs, amounting to about $6000. One person had not been aware of his hepatitis C status in time to submit a claim because he did not have regular haemophilia reviews.

Most who had received compensation recalled it as a major struggle to get what they had, largely by 'getting the run around' from ACC as they fought a 'paper war' in order to supply all the information required within the appropriate time frame. One man described it as 'like trying to get blood out of a stone', and that ACC looked upon hepatitis C as not causing any health problems: 'You have to prove that there's something wrong with you. "Why should I?" ' Another man who was unable to work due to symptoms of hepatitis C commented that attempts to get people off compensation and back to work were based on unfair criteria:

> [ACC's work capacity test] looks at physical function, so stuff like the fact that your cognitive function is not so good, that you can't predict from day to day how well you are going to be in order to work is irrelevant. If on the day they measure you they decide that physically you are capable of licking stamps and envelopes, then so be it.

Respondents were also incensed with the government's failure to accept responsibility for the 'bad blood' scandal and address compensation adequately. It was generally felt that even the compensation that some got under the old ACC Act was inadequate and that they should have received the full amount of entitlement ($27,000).

Another interviewee spoke of feeling like a 'political football' as the issue periodically came up in the media, only to die down again with no solution reached. While some people with haemophilia had spoken out publicly about the issue, some were still hesitant to disclose their hepatitis C status, much like the teenage brothers who simultaneously wanted to speak out at their unfair treatment, but wanted to maintain their confidentiality. This was a recurrent theme.

The majority interviewed had joined a legal action, commenced in April 1995, whereby people sought the full entitlement under the 1982 Act and several had joined in some of the protest events or provided media with information. The general feeling that emerged in relation to these dealings with government and ACC was that the saga had undermined their faith in the state, or as one man put it, 'it has soured my relationship with the whole system'. This sentiment was particularly significant given that people with haemophilia in general have an 'intimate reliance' on the State. Given this reliance, and the bungling of issues relating to hepatitis C by successive governments, the feelings of outrage and fears about 'what's next?' are unsurprising and an underlying feature in the lives of people with haemophilia.

When HFNZ undertook a survey of their membership in 2003 on the topic of hepatitis C to establish their members' health status and priorities for settlement, it discovered that the expectations of members had moved from compensation to the need for free access to high quality health services. Of the 189 people infected, 80 had filed a medical misadventure claim with ACC or sought compensation for loss of earnings (Carnahan 2013, 54). Only 60 people had had their claim accepted. Regional variations were evident in the numbers and proportions of claims accepted by ACC. Deaths had occurred directly as a result of hepatitis C. About 20 people had spontaneously cleared the virus. Less than 10 were in active treatment, 17 were not aware of their viral status, and more than 110 were awaiting treatment. These results were reported to the Ministry of Health at the beginning of 2004. Having collected information for each member, HFNZ pursued ACC rights on an individual basis and by January 2005 had instigated acceptance of 99 claims by providing comprehensive information and advocating on behalf of individuals. While the acceptance of those claims was a cause for celebration, the need for such vigilant advocacy by HFNZ on behalf of each individual to have each claim accepted is an indicator of the barriers experienced by people with haemophilia and hepatitis C.

HFNZ has repeated surveys of people with haemophilia and hepatitis C (Carnahan 2013, 64; Lauzon 2012). In 2011, of 189 infected, 41 had died, more than one-third of them from causes directly related to hepatitis C. Twenty-nine people had cleared the virus naturally and 58 through interferon treatment. Of the remaining 61, about half had had interferon treatment that was unsuccessful in clearing the virus. However, a new genetically targeted treatment, boceprevir, in combination with peginterferon alfa and ribavirin, which was funded from 1 September 2013, was successful for some of those with Genotype 1 who still had hepatitis C and reduced the treatment time (PHARMAC 21 August 2014). Since then, other treatment options—some of which do not require interferon and therefore do not produce such debilitating side effects—have been, and are being, developed. However, they are particularly expensive (e.g., $140,000 for one patient), and without a price reduction and funding by PHARMAC, they would be out of the reach of most New Zealanders, even when approved for use in New Zealand. In May 2016, PHARMAC announced funding for some of these new drugs.

The experience of many people with haemophilia and hepatitis C with ACC provides a salutary example of how the lack of acknowledgement of others' pain by officials of the state, running alongside a continually 'reforming' bureaucratic welfare structure, which has become divorced from the everyday practice of care (Hage 2003), increases social suffering. Hage writes about Australia but his thinking about the state and its citizens is relevant in other contexts. As he notes, affective belonging is usually left out of work on political participation. However, he proposes that one can think of societies as 'mechanisms for the distribution of hope, and that the kind of affective attachment (worrying or caring) that a society creates among its citizens is intimately connected to its capacity to distribute hope' (Hage 2003, 3). Caring is generated by an embracing society that creates hope for its citizens, understood as a disposition to embrace life. A caring state not only induces reciprocal caring but makes a cared-for citizen feel 'like a human being' (Hage 2003, 147). The reverse is more relevant to the hepatitis C situation.

The details of the hepatitis C settlement saga are complex (Carnahan 2013; Lauzon 2008) and excluded people with haemophilia in a range of ways. Some participants decided not to pursue their claim for hepatitis C because the amount available through an independence allowance was seen as 'demeaning'. Others were too sick to fight, or having already been through the process with HIV, did not want the aggravation: 'just another thing to get bitter and twisted about. I had enough things to get all bitter and twisted about. So in that respect it was an aggravation I could do without' (Man with HIV and hepatitis C).

The concept of a payout was not attractive to some people we spoke to. One young man with hepatitis C said in 2005 that he was glad that this was not how the settlement was going to be framed, because to him, a payout was tantamount to being cast adrift. He said, 'If I was to be paid out—but you see "paying out", I don't like that either, because, you see, "You're paid out, see ya! Off you go" [he laughed].' He did not want the payment of compensation to sever his ties of care from the state, nor did he see money as the answer. Instead, he concluded: 'All I'd want, if I was bad, is a hospital bed to be in, a place to be, if I was very sick from it.' A long-term relationship of care was what he was interested in.

As chapter 6 explains, a more constructive relationship finally developed between the Ministry of Health and the Foundation, ACC was side-lined, and the parties moved toward a settlement, which was achieved in principle at the end of 2006. Vocabulary around the settlement was not just about rights (and wrongs) and compensation, but about care: recognition of 'government failure in its duty of care', a settlement package about financial redress and about guarantees of good care and good treatment of hepatitis C (and haemophilia) into the future, and about partnership between HFNZ and the state.

This social suffering visited on the haemophilia community through their treatment by the multifaceted state over hepatitis C was one of the key issues that, we suggest, turned the former Haemophilia Society into a highly politicised group. Although a formal apology was not in the end forthcoming, those people who accepted the settlement finally available in 2008 received an 'expression of regret' from the Prime Minister (Lauzon 2008, 173; Park and York 2008): acknowledgement of pain at last and for some, but not all, a sense of redress and a recognition of their humanity.

Local biologies: haemophilia, HIV, and hepatitis C in international contexts

The experience of the combination of haemophilia, HIV, and hepatitis C caused crises in all the countries that used blood products for haemophilia treatment: the 'same' constellation of diseases but, at the same time, very different overall experiences. Stark differences depended on the health service, the blood supply system, the population infection rate, and the social and political contexts. For example, three countries with roughly similar population sizes, and therefore roughly similar amounts of haemophilia, are Ireland, New Zealand, and Finland. Yet Ireland had more than three times as many haemophilia patients infected with HIV as did New Zealand, which had 28. In Finland, where 90 per cent of 214 people with haemophilia were tested between 1985–9, only two people had HIV and no positive tests were returned after 1985 (Rasi *et al.* 1991).[3]

The prevalence of hepatitis C in countries like New Zealand was much higher in people who used blood products than HIV's prevalence because hepatitis C took so much longer to be identified and for the blood supply to be effectively treated. But there are major differences between countries. In the United States, it was estimated that nearly 100 per cent of people treated regularly for haemophilia were infected whereas in New Zealand at the height of the epidemic 70 per cent was the estimate. Something as basic as a low prevalence of HIV or hepatitis C in the haemophilia population is a complex outcome of a low population background infection rate, self-sufficiency in blood supply, or at least reliance on safer sources, early screening and effective treatment of donated blood, and careful monitoring and use of product (Rasi *et al.* 1991). These conditions are also outcomes of many complex, mainly social, factors. Networks and technologies of care are key here.

Despite such stark differences, there are also striking similarities in the experiences of people with haemophilia, their families, and their supporters. Extreme frustration, anger, a sense that they were not considered worth the effort to protect, social exclusion, betrayal of trust, and grief were hallmarks of the experience, constantly reiterated in interviews and in those nations where commissions of enquiry, tribunals or court cases were held, such as Canada, France, Republic of Ireland, and the United Kingdom (Archer and Willets 2009; Casteret 1992; Government of Ireland 2002; Krever 1997). But even official attention to the blood crisis created differences. People with haemophilia in New Zealand were denied such a public forum, compounding their sense of exclusion. In Iraq, there was total exclusion. People were required to detain themselves at home or forcibly incarcerated in sanitaria, deprived of their rights to work, attend school, or marry, and were told not to speak of their situation under pain of death. Their homes had notices put on them, warning people away. Even by 2006, they received no medical treatment but were paid a small benefit. A group of the Iraqi survivors, families, and the Iraq Red Crescent sued their Ministry of Health and two French and Austrian pharmaceutical companies (von Zielbauer 2006).

In some other countries, such as Taiwan, Hong Kong, and parts of Latin America, people with haemophilia discovered to their intense distress that products that were known or deemed likely to be contaminated, and therefore not used in Europe or the US, were exported by multinational pharmaceutical companies to certain countries to be 'used up' i.e., infused into citizens, as if their lives were less valuable (Bogdanich and Koli 2003).

Although anger and a sense of betrayal were part of the epidemic, the identified perpetrators were different from nation to nation. In New Zealand, as in the United Kingdom and Ireland, some parts of the national health service and certain politicians were the main focus (Archer and Willets 2009; Government of Ireland 2002; Park 2013), although some drug companies were also implicated. In other countries, such as the US or Iran, particular pharmaceutical companies that produced and sold the products were the focus; in others it was the blood service organisations, including state organisations and politicians, as in Ireland or nongovernmental organisations, such as the Red Cross in Canada (Krever 1997). And in several countries, it was a combination of these organisations and individuals, linked in a chain of culpability, such as in France (BBC News 1999; Casteret 1992)[4].

Conclusion

Viral contamination of blood products had profound effects on the haemophilia community, locally and internationally. This chapter has traced the suffering incurred by hepatitis C, from the very personal difficulties of living with a potentially life-threatening infection to the collective sense of abandonment by the state. The role of laboratory tests rather than the patients' experience of illness in granting hepatitis C the status of a diagnosis is a salutary example of how permission to be ill is achieved. Framing these personal and community experiences as local biologies of haemophilia and hepatitis C in the context of social suffering has enabled us to highlight the intertwined social, cultural, and medical elements of this predicament of haemophilia and how people's suffering is intimately linked to the state. It has also allowed insights into the New Zealand state and society, which raises moral questions of care and responsibility in the neoliberalising contexts in which these viruses developed. These issues are considered in detail in the following chapter.

Notes

1. Estimations of the numbers of New Zealanders who have hepatitis C range widely up to 60,000, but the Ministry of Health estimates there were about 50,000 living with it in 2013, whereas in 2000, the estimate was about 25,000 (Ministry of Health 2013).
2. Hepatitis C conference proceedings, 1999, Second Australasian Conference on Hepatitis C, Christchurch, New Zealand. HFNZ Archives, Christchurch.
3. We benefitted from reference to en.m.wikipedia.org 'Contaminated haemophilia blood products', and from this were able to retrieve archived news articles.
4. At publication, the official United Kingdom government inquiry, led by Sir Brian Langstaff, into infected blood was beginning, see www.infectedbloodinquiry.org.uk

References

Alter, H.J., and H.G. Klein. 2008. 'The Hazards of Blood Transfusion in Historical Perspective'. *Blood* 7 (112):2617–26.

N.J., Archer, The Rt Hon and J. Willets. 2009. 'Independent Public Inquiry Report on NHS Supplied Contaminated Blood and Blood products'. https://haemophiliascotland.files.wordpress.com/2014/11/76_lord-archer-report.pdf (last accessed 11 Nov, 2018).

Auckland Star. 1984. 'Blood Tainted by AIDS'. *Auckland Star*, November 5.

BBC News. 1999. 'World: Europe Blood Scandal Ministers Walk Free'. *BBC News*, March 8. http://news.bbc.co.uk/2/hi/europe/293367.stm (last accessed 11 Nov, 2018).

Berry, E., and P.J. Wyld. 1983. 'Haemophilia, Blood Products and AIDS'. *New Zealand Medical Journal* 96 (744):986.

Bogdanich, W., and E. Koli, 2003. '2 Paths of Bayer drug in 80's: Riskier One Steered Overseas'. *The New York Times* 22 May.

Carnahan, M.J. 2013. *Allies or Enemies: How Those Needing Help Learned to Help Themselves in the Face of Bad Blood*. Christchurch: Haemophilia Foundation of New Zealand.

Casteret, A.-M. 1992. *L'Affaire du Sang*. Paris: Éditions La Découverte.

Chen, S.L. and T.R. Morgan. 2006. 'The Natural History of Hepatitis C Virus (HCV) Infection'. *International Journal of Medical Sciences* 3 (2):47–52.

Choo, Q-L., G. Kuo, A.J. Weiner, L.R. Overby, D.W. Bradley, and M. Houghton. 1989. 'Isolation of a cDNA Clone Derived from a Blood-borne Non-A, Non-B Viral Hepatitis Genome'. *Science* 244 (4902):359–62.

Crossen, K.A., C.R. Brunton, E. Plumridge and W. Jang. 1999. 'The Experiences of People Living with Hepatitis C.' Paper presented to the Second Australasian Conference on Hepatitis C, Hepatitis C: The Evolving Epidemic, Christchurch, August 171–9.

Daly, R., with P. Cunningham. 2003. *A Case of Bad Blood*. Dublin: Poolbeg Press.

Department of Health. 1992. 'Inquiry into Matters Relating to the Safety of Blood Products in New Zealand'. Wellington: Department of Health.

Dickson, N., and C. Paul. 1996. 'HIV Infection and AIDS in New Zealand: A Public Health Report'. In *Intimate Details & Vital Statistics: AIDS, Sexuality and the Social Order in New Zealand*, edited by P. Davis, 13–30. Auckland: Auckland University Press.

Garrett, L., and S. Conrad. 2001. 'Quality of life: Are People Living with Chronic Hepatitis C Getting Enough?' *Australian Hepatitis Chronicle* 8:4–8.

Gifford, S. 1999. 'Bad Livers, Bad Blood, Bad Women? New Challenges for Healing the Illness'. Paper presented to the Second Australasian Conference on Hepatitis C, Hepatitis C: The Evolving Epidemic. Christchurch, August 17–19.

Government of Ireland [Lindsay Tribunal]. 2002. 'Report of the Tribunal of Inquiry into the Infection with HIV and Hepatitis C of Persons with Haemophilia and Related Matters'. Dublin: Stationery Office.

Hage, G. 2003. *Against Paranoid Nationalism: Searching for Hope in a Shrinking Society.* Annadale, NSW: Pluto Press and Merlin.

Howden-Chapman P. 1994. 'Blood Ties: Accountability for Blood Quality in New Zealand'. *Health Policy* 27 (1):35–51.

Keshavjee, S., S. Weiser, and A. Kleinman. 2001. 'Medicine Betrayed: Hemophilia Patients and HIV in the US'. *Social Science and Medicine* 53:1081–94.

Kleinman, A., V. Das, and M. Lock. 1997. 'Introduction'. In *Social Suffering*, edited by Kleinman, A., V. Das, and M. Lock, ix-xxvii. Berkeley: University of California Press.

Krever, H. 1997. 'Final Report: Commission of Inquiry on the Blood System in Canada'. Ottawa: The Commission.

Lauzon, C. 2008. *Still Standing: Haemophilia Foundation of New Zealand 1958–2008.* Christchurch: Haemophilia Foundation of New Zealand Inc.

———. 2012. '"Like a Curse": Outcomes of the "New Zealand 2011 People with Haemophilia and Hepatitis C Survey"'. *Haemophilia* 18 (Suppl.3):83.

Lee, C. 1999. 'Hepatitis C Infection and its Management'. *Haemophilia* 5:365–70.

McLean, J. 1999. 'It's Personal'. Paper presented to the Second Australasian Conference on Hepatitis C, Hepatitis C: The Evolving Epidemic, Christchurch, August 17–19.

Ministry of Health. 2013.'Hepatitis C'. https://www.health.govt.nz/your-health/conditions-and-treatments/diseases-and-illnesses/hepatitis-c (last accessed 11 Nov, 2018).

Mol, A. 2002. *The Body Multiple: Ontology in Medical Practice.* Durham: Duke University Press.

Nettleton, S. 2006. '"I just want permission to be ill": Towards a sociology of medically unexplained symptoms'. *Social Science & Medicine* 62:1167–78.

Park, J. 2013. 'Painful exclusion: Hepatitis C in the New Zealand Haemophilia Community'. In *Senses and Citizenships: Embodying Political Life*, edited by S. Trnka, C. Dureau, and J. Park, 221–41. New York: Routledge.

Park, J., and D. York. 2008. *The Social Ecology of New Technologies and Haemophilia in New Zealand: 'A Bleeding Nuisance' Revisited.* Research in Anthropology & Linguistics 8. Auckland: Department of Anthropology, University of Auckland. https://researchspace.auckland.ac.nz/handle/2292/4534 (last accessed 11 Nov, 2018).

Parsons, T. 1951. *The Social System.* Glencoe Il: The Free Press.

PHARMAC. 2014. 'Genetic Markers Being Used to Target New Oral Hepatitis C Drug'. August 21. www.pharmac.health.nz/news/media-2014-08-21-hepc (last accessed 11 Nov, 2018).

Rasi, V., E. Ikkala, F. Myllylä, and H.R. Nevanlinna. 1991. 'Low Prevalence of Antibodies Against Human Immunodeficiency Virus in Finnish Haemophiliacs'. *Vox Sanguinis* 60 (3):159–61.

Renault, P.F., J.H. Hoofnagle, Y. Park, K.P. Mullen, M. Peters, D.B. Jones, V. Rustgi, and E.A. Jones. 1987. 'Psychiatric Complications of Long-term Interferon Alfa Therapy'. *Archives of Internal Medicine* 147:1577–80.

Resnik, S. 1999. *Blood Saga: Hemophilia, AIDS, and the Survival of a Community.* Berkeley: University of California Press.

Shipley, Rt Hon J. 1992. *New Zealand Parliamentary Debates* (Hansard) 3455, April 24.

Taylor, G., and M.P. Power. 2011. *Risk, Science and Blood: Politics, HIV, Hepatitis and Haemophilia in Ireland.* Galway: ARAN, Access to Research at NUI Galway. http://hdl.handle.net/10379/2547 (last accessed 11 Nov, 2018).

TVNZ. 1992. *Tonight* Programme. Television One. November 16.

von Zielbauer, P. 2006. 'Iraqis Infected by HIV-Tainted Blood Try New Tool: A Law Suit'. *The New York Times*, September 4.

Woodfield, D.G. 1991. 'Hepatitis C Virus (HCV) Infections in New Zealand'. *Gastroenterologia Japonica* 26 (Supplement 3):189–91.

6 Joint action

Asserting rights, inclusion, and equity through voluntary association

From rights to equity

The golden era of blood-derived concentrates came to an abrupt end in 1983 with the discovery that HIV was transmitted through the blood supply. This crisis, which was soon followed by the discovery of widespread hepatitis C infection, had a traumatic effect on individuals, families, and the entire hae-mophilia community (chapter 5). In this chapter, in contrast, we turn to collec-tive political action led by the Haemophilia Society (NZHS) in response to the crisis, resulting eventually in the ground-breaking hepatitis C settlement from the state. This decade-and-a-half of lobbying also laid the foundations for successful championing of national standards of haemophilia care, improving care in some parts of the country that were poorly served. In turn, this work contributed to the establishment of the National Haemophilia Management Group (NHMG) in 2006 to oversee all haemophilia care. These changes in the networks of care influenced the local biology of haemophilia: the political effects were embodied in daily lives.

Neoliberal reforms were deeply implicated in viral politics from the mid-1980s, as Taylor and Power (2011, 6) noted in relation to Ireland:

> Blood is a political issue precisely because it touches upon matters that are at the heart of Irish democracy: deliberation upon the role of public and private sector provision in welfare services, the power of multinational pharmaceutical companies, the impact of regulatory reform on science.

Taylor and Power contend that conservative politics of the New Right, particularly governmental fiscal constraint and the reduction of regulatory red tape, made way for multinational pharmaceutical companies to make key decisions about blood safety. Intervention to protect the safety of the public blood supply could only be justified on the grounds of scientifically proven risk, and even then it should be considered 'proportional' to market considerations. We analyse the same era in New Zealand, but shift the lens to examine how neoliberal discourses and practices were employed and subverted by a group of volunteers to exert collective political influence.

After nearly three decades of neoliberal reforms that had devolved governance of healthcare to the regional scale, the decision to centralise funding allocation and strategic direction of haemophilia care in 2006 denoted a landmark change. NZHS, by now renamed the Haemophilia Foundation of New Zealand (HFNZ), worked with medical associates and authorities to implement a system that has successfully improved quality in care and regionally equitable treatment standards. Furthermore, the new national governance structure was subsequently replicated for other high-cost conditions, suggesting that HFNZ shifted what is considered 'normal' in policy practices of participatory governance and regionalised decision-making.

Years of political lobbying transformed NZHS into a politically astute national foundation, with some paid staff and an echelon of dedicated, well-informed, if somewhat battle-weary, members. We examine narratives of differences in standards of care to reveal a strong sense of injustice that drove HFNZ's collective political action. We trace HFNZ's interactions and contestations with the state that shaped the association into an extremely 'active citizen', and one that made a considerable difference to the institutional context that determines what haemophilia is like for people with the condition and their families.

In a political context that favoured public engagement and inclusion at the local scale, we show how HFNZ effectively translated neoliberal ideology to challenge structural inequalities and shape governance of haemophilia care. Following Rose and Novas (2005), we contend that there was no single logic to explain how HFNZ achieved these outcomes. We show the constellation of historical, political, ethical, and moral forms that shaped policies, with a focus on contestation by a voluntary association that would not take no for an answer. As active citizens working in new governance spaces, HFNZ were part of the very inventiveness (Rose 1999) of neoliberalism. Larner and Craig (2005) observe that New Zealand community activists can find themselves adopting contradictory and compromising subject positions in their efforts to influence neoliberal policy agendas. However, HFNZ's version of active citizenship was somewhat different. HFNZ moved between alliance, contestation, and opposition to the state, based on trial and error, opportunism, and sheer determination. Rather than being an active citizen in the neoliberal sense as an individual who energetically pursues personal fulfilment and undertakes incessant calculations to enable this to be achieved (Miller and Rose 2008 [1992], 82), HFNZ worked collectively as a social citizen with powers and responsibility derived from its membership. It used that political position to turn governmental strategies of calculation, documentation, and evaluation back on the state to create an equitable system of care for all people with haemophilia. We examine HFNZ's subjectivity as fluid and involving 'a continuous process of experimentation—inner, familial, medical, and political … [while it] also contains creativity' (Biehl 2005, 137) to stimulate opportunities to exert political influence and avoid compromising itself.

We trace the 'rough and ready assemblages of forces' (Rose 1999, 280) that shaped policies, health outcomes, and HFNZ itself.

The chapter includes two related topics: the emergence of the Haemophilia Foundation as an engaged citizen responding to the discovery of viral contamination of the blood supply; and collective political action resulting in significant changes to the governance of haemophilia care. First, we go back in time to the establishment of NZHS in the peak of New Zealand's welfare-state era.

Emergence of the Haemophilia Society

From the time the Haemophilia Society was established in 1958, its membership included politicians, clinicians, the pharmaceutical industry and business people, along with people with haemophilia and their families. This all-embracing membership was likely due to an understanding that broad collaboration was needed to improve this life-threatening condition. Over the years the Society became a support and advocacy network run by volunteers, providing and coordinating mutual support and information for people with haemophilia and their families and advocating for improved treatment.

A Medical Advisory Committee was created to sit alongside the Society to contribute expertise and advice on medical issues. This close association with clinicians has supported the Society in their endeavour to be knowledgeable, current with emergent issues, and able to partner with physicians to advocate for quality care. Over the years, the Society also built strong links with haemophilia associations in other countries, including the World Federation of Hemophilia, formed in 1963. NZHS engaged shortly after and became an official member in 1975 when its first delegate attended World Congress (Lauzon 2008).

As early as 1974, NZHS volunteers were advocating the need for a comprehensive haemophilia care centre, thought to be 'only a dream' at that time but one that 'doctors and the hospital Board' needed to be convinced of, according to John Davy, secretary of NZHS (reprinted 2001). This may have been the first instance of the Society successfully advocating with its Medical Advisory Committee for improved haemophilia care, as the first such centre was established in Auckland in 1975 (Lauzon 2008). In contrast, NZHS's advocacy for a fractionation plant in New Zealand, which would produce the replacement clotting factors needed for treatment from blood donated by New Zealanders, was not successful and had significant implications when viral contaminants were discovered in imported blood products in the 1980s.

NZHS emerged at a time when health care and education were mostly free, and there was a strong societal view that the state had a duty of care towards citizens. Economic prosperity and high standards of living, relative to the rest of the world, contributed to a strong national discourse of egalitarianism (Shirley 1990). As we outlined in Chapter 1, despite social differentiation and inequality within New Zealand, the idea that everyone has the same rights as everyone else to fair treatment also shaped HFNZ's expectations for fair and quality treatment by the state. The story of NZHS and HFNZ provides further evidence for Fischer's (2012) thesis that fairness and natural justice are key social values in New Zealand. The concept of fairness was shown to be a powerful rhetorical tool.

NZHS and its members have long been recognised as experts on issues related to blood supply and haemophilia care. This recognition is partly due to the nature of haemophilia. People with haemophilia and their families develop a high level of expertise in their own rare and life-threatening condition and their treatment needs. We also observed that as people learn to deal with haemophilia, they develop dispositions that enable them to be persistent but diplomatic with authority figures, inclined to a partnership approach, adept at managing risk, and flexible and stoic in the face of adversity. This cultural capital helped shape (and was consequently shaped by) advocacy processes, in particular, people's expectations that they be included in decisions that affected their lives.

The haemophilia population is small and strongly networked through formal and informal ties between families and individuals. People with haemophilia saw this network as biological and social, mutually supportive and essential to getting by, given the severity of the condition, its rarity, and the consequent lack of expertise on haemophilia amongst most health professionals. The intimate links and mutual support between individuals and families were very evident during ethnographic fieldwork. Field notes collated as the researchers travelled between cities, provincial centres, and rural towns are full of references to these interconnections between interviewees. For example, from Kathryn's field notes in 1995 as she drove thousands of kilometres around the South Island visiting families with haemophilia:

> John's the uncle of young Peter that I interviewed last week; Mike's one of three brothers with haemophilia, he said I talked to his oldest brother a week ago; before I arrived, Lorna (interviewee) had been talking on the phone to Dianne (who I interviewed yesterday) about a problem bleed that her son was having and passed on her regards.

NZHS emerged as a grassroots organisation within this interconnected community. At the Society gatherings we attended in 1994 and 1995, such as family camps or AGMs, it was common to see haematologists on warm and friendly terms with whole families including wives, siblings, or parents of people with haemophilia, and uncles and cousins whom they may also have treated. Likewise, some drug company representatives were on a first-name basis with many. Men on crutches, mobility scooters, or in wheelchairs were a common sight. Daughters and nieces of some of these men often watched attentively, building up their knowledge of life with haemophilia. At family camps, parents talked incessantly about their children, like any group of parents, but here the talk also included haemophilia: how to detect a joint 'bleed', when to have a daughter tested for her carrier status, how to divert a boy away from rugby, how to respond to judgemental stares at their 'bruised banana' of a child while out in public, and the like. For many families, this was their one opportunity a year to be with a group of people who really knew what it was like to live with haemophilia and to have informal chats with haematologists and other specialists, so they made the most of it. These interactions also helped build relationships and networks that could be brought into use at later times. The strong sense of solidarity between people with haemophilia was to influence the ways that NZHS volunteers operated.

Responding to our initial questionnaire in 1994, when asked if they were members of NZHS, 60 respondents made additional, unsolicited positive comments about the Society (including voluntary and professional services) e.g., stating that it was 'worthwhile', 'good for newly diagnosed', 'approachable', 'wonderful', 'very supportive', 'excellent'. NZHS volunteers expressed a strong sense of the vulnerability of the haemophilia population and saw themselves as 'here for the long haul'; actors with the greatest interest in getting quality outcomes.

With a long history of working collectively for the benefit of the haemophilia population, including two and three generations in some families, NZHS volunteers had the trust and respect of the membership that they would work on their behalf. They also had experience of successfully lobbying collectively. Over the years, NZHS continued to advocate for improved blood safety and treatment options, always assuming that they were entitled to be involved in government decision-making processes that affected them and that working in partnership with authorities was an effective approach.

Viral politics

In December 1984, NZHS released a special issue newsletter warning that a batch of the blood product used to treat factor IX deficiency contained an HIV-related antibody and other earlier batches might have been contaminated. As described in chapter 5, this news threw the haemophilia community into a state of shock and despair that was to pervade their lives for some years. It was also the start of a new role for the Society of fighting to ensure rapid and adequate responses from the range of state agencies involved in blood and health services. How to be effective in this role was something that was not immediately apparent, and was learned through bitter experience.

In this section, we explore how HFNZ positioned itself and approached collective action related to viral contaminants, moving from a 'working together' (with health authorities) approach toward vigilant observation and open contestation, then an 'active citizen' approach, and finally, when all else failed, utilising tactics of resistance (see Figure 6.1).

Working with Govt	Watchdog Contestation	Will to Justice	Active Citizen	Tactics of Resistance
- HIV: Lobbying to secure safety of blood supply - Partnership with the state	- HCV: Lobbying to secure safety of blood supply & ACC - Rights to apology & compensation - Public protests - Class action - Submissions	- Mobilise collective action - Court media & politicians - Safe space to strategise - Support ACC claims & submissions	- Strategic reversal - Survey - Distill issues into sound bites - One person, one issue - Negotiate a settlement	- When all else fails... - Threaten politician's reputation - Hardball negotiation

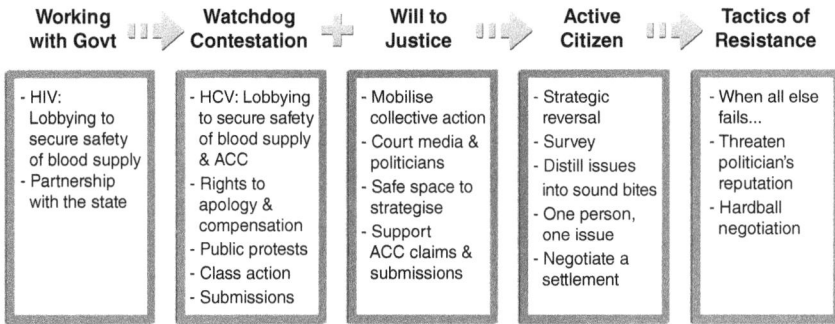

Figure 6.1 Haemophilia Society's changes in tactics.

Working with government: lobbying and partnership 1983–90

Within two days of the media release by the Auckland Blood Service that some of New Zealand's blood products were contaminated with HIV, NZHS volunteers had commenced pressuring the Minister of Health, Rt Hon Dr Michael Bassett, to introduce measures to protect the safety of the national blood supply. Dr Bassett moved quickly (Carnahan 2013, 17). Unlike their American counterparts who were hesitant to relinquish faith in concentrates that had given such improvements to quality of life (Schmidt 2011), NZHS volunteers suddenly found themselves advocating on life-and-death issues to sequester those concentrates or to make them safe. The Society recognised that they were in a unique position of having intimate knowledge of treatment and blood bank systems, and extensive networks with Health Department officials, blood banks, medical staff, and international patient organisations. Again this differed to the United States, France, Japan, and Canada where no influential group of recipients of blood products existed (Schmidt 2011). NZHS volunteers also had a strong expectation, based on years of advocacy, that they would be listened to by government officials. They worked with their Medical Advisory Committee to lobby to ensure the blood supply was made safe. Despite their best efforts, 28 people with haemophilia contracted HIV in New Zealand. Infection came from blood concentrates made by CSL Laboratories, using New Zealand and Australian blood donations.

Success in securing the eventual safety of the national blood supply was hard won, and each issue demanded enormous effort. The responsibility these volunteers shouldered was no doubt well beyond anything they might have anticipated when they were elected to voluntary committee positions on NZHS. Only a highly knowledgeable, extremely motivated, and well-networked association of volunteers could have worked on so many fronts at the same time, and to good effect. They became extremely active citizens making use of their knowledge and networks to protect the health of all New Zealanders. Had they not been so active it is likely the blood supply would have remained unsafe for longer: no other grouping had such a vested interest and capacity to act. It demonstrates that NZHS was able to exert influence at critical times through collective internal strategising and with their Medical Advisory Committee. NZHS volunteers also worked behind the scenes to support the membership in coming to terms with the discovery of HIV and AIDS, to challenge the practice of 'haemophiliacs' being labelled as a risk group (rather than 'people infected by blood and blood products') (Park *et al.* 1995, 37), and to counter or prevent stigmatising in the media and the community.

Because NZHS was resourced by volunteers, it was able to criticise and lobby government. This was in stark contrast to haemophilia associations in some other parts of the world that were closely aligned with pharmaceutical companies and have been widely criticised for not advocating on behalf of people with haemophilia, or worse, recommending people use products that the association knew to be contaminated or refusing to support claims for compensation (Kirp 1999).

Our research interviews 1994–5 suggested that participants were mostly satisfied that further avoidable infection with HIV was averted by the measures that were adopted as a result of NZHS's and the Medical Advisory Committee's advocacy. This included heat treatment (to 60°C) of all blood concentrates by January 1985.[1] Government agencies were judged to have acted quickly to ensure blood safety in response to HIV and AIDS. The haemophilia community became aware that by comparison with many other countries, blood contamination had resulted in a relatively low incidence of HIV in people with haemophilia in New Zealand, in contrast to parts of the world that were reliant on American concentrates sourced from paid-donor collection. In Spain, for example, 41 per cent of people with haemophilia tested positive for HIV by 1992, closely followed by Japan at 40 per cent, France at 38 per cent, and the United Kingdom at 34 per cent (Farrell 2006; Schmidt 2011). As noted in the previous chapter, Ireland, which has a similar size population as New Zealand, continued to use non-heat-treated concentrates until June 1986, and as a result, over 100 people with haemophilia (25 per cent of the haemophilia treatment population) contracted HIV (Taylor and Power 2011).[2]

The Haemophilia Society's archives show the tremendous amount of time and effort volunteers exerted to ensure appropriate steps were taken to protect the national blood supply, such as gathering the latest information and writing letters to government officials and ministers. They were repeatedly faced with institutional inertia and other barriers. For example, NZHS tried and failed to have random donor cryoprecipitate phased out immediately because of the risk of viral contamination. They also failed to get super-heat-treated (to 80°C) blood products introduced and to get NZHS representation on BTAC.

Even after the safety of the blood supply was secured against HIV, the volunteers' role was far from over. Volunteers became immersed in supporting families to access compensation from ACC. A national no-fault ACC system had been in place since 1974.[3] From 1987 the Society fought for equitable and adequate compensation, often on a case-by-case basis, while supporting those individuals in their dealings with ACC. As with securing the safety of the blood supply, achieving equitable compensation involved activities on several fronts. The volunteers advocated on disputes with ACC over the degree of progression of disease since this influenced the amount of compensation given. The NZHS also funded legal action in some cases, and prepared and presented submissions to government ministries,[4] the New Zealand Law Commission, and ACC review hearings (Carnahan 2013). This was exhausting work, but, in the face of crisis, this voluntary association mobilised collectively to demand justice.

New professional role for the Society

In response to this viral crisis in the haemophilia community, NZHS attracted funding from a national AIDS taskforce to employ an outreach worker to provide support to people with haemophilia and HIV. This denoted a change in NZHS's role beyond a solely voluntary association to being an organisation of volunteers and professional staff. Volunteers continued in elected positions of president, secretary, newsletter editor, and regional committee members. The outreach worker took up a large part of the support role for people with HIV in their dealings with ACC and other government agencies. This support proved so valuable that the service was later extended through public funding to all people with haemophilia, and the number of outreach workers increased over the years to four. From 1992, the Society also employed an administrator on a part-time basis, funded by the Lotteries Board.

This arrangement of community organisations becoming the employers of professional health workers was promoted by a National Government, and was a precursor to what became a widespread governance model in the health service a decade later. Contrary to the critique that such a partially publicly funded role inevitably silences political action by the group (Miller and Rose 2008 [1996]), NZHS retained their ability to contest policies or decisions related to haemophilia and treatment issues by carefully directing public funding toward specific roles or projects. New Zealand has just one voluntary association for people with haemophilia, and therefore can speak with one powerful voice for the nation's haemophilia population. This is in stark contrast to the United States, for example, where memberships are large but divided between different associations, blood products are locally sourced and produced, and associations are organised by medical professionals and funded by pharmaceutical companies (Kirp 1999).

Watchdog tactics in extraordinary times: contestation and lobbying 1990–2003

In 1989, hepatitis C was characterised, and blood-screening for this virus was developed. When we began our research in 1994, hepatitis C was known to have a long incubation period and the medical profession considered it relatively benign. Over time, this view changed and it is now known that 10–15 per cent of those with chronic infection develop serious cirrhosis of the liver and in some cases liver cancer and other life threatening conditions (Chen and Morgan 2006).

Screening of donated blood became routine in Australia in 1990 but was not fully implemented in New Zealand until February 1993 (Carnahan 2013, 28 & 36; Park *et al.* 1995). Among the participants in our 1994–5 study who had moderate or severe haemophilia 57 per cent (58 people) reported that they had contracted hepatitis C, and 84 of the total of 193 participants (44 per cent). Yet the haemophilia population was effectively excluded from the limited measures taken by government to rectify and compensate those affected due mainly to stipulations about timing. These included both the time limit for lodging claims and the impossibility of people knowing for sure when they had been infected. Even in 1995, 12 per cent of the participants did not know their hepatitis C status (Park *et al.* 1995, 40). The felt injustice, the increasing health concerns of those starting to become ill as a consequence of chronic infection with the virus, and dealing with the ambivalence of some specialists about this disease, were to occupy the efforts of the NZHS and HFNZ for the next decade-and-a-half.

Initially, NZHS worked collaboratively with other actors to ensure the blood supply was safe, as they had done in the past. The Society also employed more outreach workers to help provide extra care for those affected. A hepatitis C subcommittee of elected members was formed. These volunteers were educated, knowledgeable about the health system, and had a long personal and family history of involvement in NZHS and in self and family advocacy to access quality haemophilia treatment. They were also either self-employed or retired, and therefore had some control over their time.

The NZHS provided a space of interaction where volunteers could come together to share information and strategise before lobbying government, as in the case of HIV. When delays in the introduction of adequate blood safety measures became evident in the early 1990s, NZHS again chose to undertake lobbying at a governance level, protecting salaried staff from involvement, because, as one participant explained it, 'they can't afford to get off side with the Ministry of Health'.

The Society's traditional approach of working in collaboration with government agencies and writing letters to the Ministry was proving ineffective, as was making the issues public. When confronted by media statements about their failures to introduce adequate measures to protect the safety of blood products, government ministers inevitably denied all knowledge of the inadequacies and assured the public that the problem would be investigated and fixed. Even when promises were finally made by the Minister of Health that adequate measures would be instigated, NZHS learned this did not necessarily mean such promises would be implemented.

This was a new era in health care and accident compensation in New Zealand. Volunteers found they had to adopt a hyper-vigilant watchdog approach, continually challenging delays in introducing super-heat-treated (to 80°C) blood products, in screening blood donors, testing blood, and in notification of diagnoses.[5] Minister of Health, Helen Clark, diverted the responsibility for these actions to the Area Health Boards, despite the fact that the AHBs did not deal with manufacturing standards for blood products. NZHS then made direct recommendations to BTAC, which in turn recommended the introduction of hepatitis C antibody screening of all blood donations collected in New Zealand to the Director General of Health. This recommendation was supported by an influential network of Regional Transfusion Directors, the Communicable Disease Control Advisory Committee, and a leading article in the *New Zealand Medical Journal* (Tasman-Jones 1990). But it was July 1992 before testing of factor VIII was implemented, and people with haemophilia B had to wait until February 1993 before factor IX was screened and tested. This occurred at a time when political appetite for decentralisation of decision making and resource allocation was at its peak. The hepatitis C debacle is a stark example of how this can lead to disastrous results.

For NZHS, all notions of working with the government ceased when it emerged that senior health managers chose to continue using blood products that were known to be infected with hepatitis C. These people were never held to account in any way for their actions. Their decision was based on the belief that the virus was not serious, and, as Ministry Principal Medical Advisor stated on the *Tonight* television programme, ACC would compensate (TVNZ 1992; see Chapter 5).

> In Australia, health authorities had to screen to protect themselves from legal actions. But here ... we were protected because ACC would cover those who became contaminated.

Haemophilia Society volunteers reeled at this admission, but it did help confirm their suspicions that money came first for government. Changes to the ACC Act in 1992 prevented this compensation from being awarded, adding to the outrage at this statement and further fuelling the Society's determination to get justice for those affected.

Suddenly we were on the outside of the tent

As in the case of HIV, securing the safety of the national blood supply was just the first step. NZHS had a much longer fight on their hands—achieving equitable ACC compensation for what the Society referred to as 'victims of tainted blood'.

The Society argued strongly, over many years, that the Ministry of Health had failed in its duty of care to protect people with haemophilia from viral contamination in the blood supply and that those infected were therefore entitled to compensation and an apology. However, the revision of accident compensation provisions through the introduction of the Accident Compensation and Rehabilitation Act 1992, effective from 1 April 1992, had huge implications for people who had contracted hepatitis C through the blood supply. As we detailed in chapter 5, most people with haemophilia were excluded. Furthermore, over time the Haemophilia Society found that ACC legislation and accompanying regulations were interpreted in different ways around the country, leading to a strong sense of injustice.

The Haemophilia Society found that its customary approach of working with government agencies and in a mediation role between its membership and the state was no longer possible, as one participant explained:

> We had reasonably close connections with the Ministry of Health, and then suddenly we were on the outside of the tent, because they decided to break it up into all these different categories of where people deal with it … for example, the Infectious Diseases Committee … IV Drug (users) Committee … the blood transfusion people. And cynically I have to say that that was deliberate … the Ministry pushed them apart so they didn't correlate information or strategies.

Nevertheless, the NZHS was able to draw on existing alliances with haematologists, the World Federation of Hemophilia and other haemophilia associations, and formed new alliances, such as with the AIDS Foundation, Hepatitis C Support Group, and the Coalition for medically fragile families, all of which were nongovernmental organisations that were very involved in lobbying on similar issues to the Haemophilia Society. With the support of these allies, and faced with apparent indifference from the government, the Society adopted a much more militant role, positioning themselves in opposition to government.

Will to Justice: demanding rights to fair compensation

The Society felt they had 'no option' but to undertake escalating public action aimed at pressuring politicians to resolve the issue. These actions included public protests, making submissions, taking a class action against ACC, and even making a complaint of criminal nuisance against previous Ministers of Health, Helen Clark (by now Prime Minister) and Simon Upton. None of these tactics had the desired effect.

At this time when a right-of-centre government was pursuing free market policies and advocating reduced state reliance and greater individual responsibility, this 'reciprocity principle' (Standing 2010) was turned back on the state by HFNZ, albeit with limited success at that time. One person identified a mismatch between government discourses and practices of individual rights and responsibilities:

> I am offended by the government not accepting its responsibilities ... it makes my blood boil ... the government tells us that we should row our own boats, take responsibility for ourselves, but the government is not taking responsibility for their own errors and areas of responsibility. I expect at least an apology. (Interview, young man, 1995)

In relation to hepatitis C, NZHS was also advocating rights and responsibilities at this time: rights to recognition for the betrayal of the haemophilia community in knowingly allowing contaminated products to be administered; rights to adequate treatment for hepatitis C; rights to an apology; and rights to fair recompense. This insistence on rights, pursued through a class action being taken on behalf of individuals, reflected a global rights discourse that highlighted an individual's rights relative to the state.

NZHS framed the state's obligations as a duty of care, meaning a duty to provide a standard of reasonable care while performing any acts that could harm others. All the actors assumed that the state had a duty of care toward people with haemophilia, and citizens had a right to a duty of care by the state and its agents. The battle was over whether the state had failed in its duty of care, and if so, whether individuals should be compensated, echoing situations where the state does not assume a duty of care toward certain individuals. Rabeharisoa (2006), for example, describes political activism initiated in the 1950s in France by a Muscular Dystrophy patient organisation to have the condition acknowledged as a disease, to initiate research to find a cure for the disease, and to ensure that individuals affected by the disease were acknowledged as full citizens and deserving of care.

In New Zealand, in the case of hepatitis C the main 'villains' were politicians who, as elected representatives, were responsible for health service failures, some health bureaucrats, and ACC's failure to reach a settlement with people with haemophilia. The villains were not pharmaceutical companies who supplied the blood products. Again, this contrasted with other parts of the world where people with haemophilia sought compensation from drug companies, and in some cases were successful (Kirp 1999).

Claims about failures in duty of care were closely linked to circulating global discourses of rights, with the focus on rights of individuals. The rise of human rights claims among international aid agencies and other NGOs evident since the 1990s has been critiqued as rhetorical repackaging to divert attention from structural inequalities. As Uvin identified, this amounted to a redefinition of the nature of the problem, a 'move from needs to rights, and from charity to duties. It also implies an increased focus on accountability' (2010, 170), and is therefore closely linked to emergent neo-liberal constructs of 'good governance'.

During the first phase of our study in the mid-1990s, the shift from charity to duties was particularly relevant to the haemophilia community, as gifted blood products were being gradually replaced by recombinant products. Many children with haemophilia had become consumers of recombinant products from multinational pharmaceutical companies. Access to safe and secure supply of treatment products was becoming linked to consumer rights, with notions of the products being 'fit for purpose' deriving from consumer legislation, and to responsibilities of citizen-consumers to use the products prudently. This shift was significant as it also shifted lines of responsibilities. While NZHS claimed bio-political rights to compensation and treatment based on their vulnerability and right to be protected from harm, these rights were not clearly evident in legal terms.

This time of our initial study, which coincided with the start of NZHS's struggle over hepatitis C, was a period of great change. Then, gifted blood was still the basis of most treatment products. Only young children who had had no exposure to viral contamination were treated with recombinant products that were gifted from drug companies, although these products were not yet part of government purchasing policy. So while parents of young children grappled with their rights and responsibilities as consumers of gifted and highly sought-after recombinant products, most of the adult haemophilia population struggled with the fallout from being recipients of products from gifted blood.

Gifted blood brought a symbolic weight into the moral discourses related to the hepatitis C battle. The actions of successive governments indicated that recipients of the life-giving properties of gifted blood were not entitled to compensation, even if in this case these products were also life-taking. This suggests that the health service was based on the principle of 'all care, no responsibility' rather than a fundamental duty of care for all citizens. In response to media attention, the Department of Health directed attention to advisory committees and the blood transfusion service, and so it was not surprising that an inquiry in 1992 commissioned by the Department failed to clearly locate where responsibility lay for the hepatitis C debacle (Department of Health 1992).

NZHS portrayed people with haemophilia who contracted hepatitis C as victims, but did not emphasise their status as 'innocent' victims, downplaying negative comparisons with other high-risk groups such as gay men and drug users. This differed considerably to the United States where the haemophilia population overtly differentiated themselves from other high-risk groups and promoted the view of people with haemophilia as innocent victims (Kirp 1999; Resnik 1999). Haemophilia Society members active in local protests stated that while public protests were emotionally satisfying and helped raise public and media knowledge about the issues, they did not bring desired political results. Nevertheless, they continued trying to come up with inventive ways of raising the profile of the hepatitis C issue and force a resolution.

From Society to Foundation

In 1999, the New Zealand Haemophilia Society was renamed the Haemophilia Foundation of New Zealand. A National Council was established comprising president, vice presidents (two), treasurer, secretary, and delegates from the four new branches, Northern, Midland, Central, and Southern (NZHS 1998, 4). This structure enabled greater connection between more isolated branches, and therefore a greater capacity to work collectively to contest injustices.

In some ways, the association remained much the same. The services of the (paid) outreach workers, the provision of newsletters and educational camps and workshops continued to be the most public aspects of the Foundation activities. Its membership continued to be a diverse mix of individuals and families, associates, corporations, friends, patrons, and life members. Positions on the National Council and special committees continued to be voluntary, meaning they could continue with lobbying and advocacy,[6] leaving paid staff to undertake the day-to-day support of the membership. The part-time administrator position created in 1992 grew and changed into a Chief Executive position in 2003.

The shift toward a more corporate model for the Foundation reflected their increased budget for supporting the membership. Since 1997, fundraising had been done by a fundraising company operated by a man with haemophilia (Lauzon 2008), resulting in the doubling of their annual budget and relieving volunteers from the arduous task of raising money. As a result, HFNZ was able to offer much greater support to its membership. Government funding continued to be exclusively for the outreach workers to provide support for families and individuals.

HFNZ appointed several multinational drug companies as sustaining patrons, and any money these companies donated was carefully channelled to specific projects. By welcoming several companies as patrons, the Foundation did not favour, nor was it beholden to, any particular one. This strategy was a carefully considered response to the commodified environment created by the highly visible multinational companies.

An active citizen approach

In 2003, HFNZ's hepatitis C team shifted tack in their efforts to achieve justice for all people with haemophilia who had been excluded from earlier hepatitis C settlement deals. Recognising that demanding rights from an oppositional position was not getting the desired results, they now adopted an active citizen persona. This involved a staged, proactive approach to pressuring politicians in the lead-up to the general election in September 2005. HFNZ retained its watchdog role but, like a good active citizen, also sought to work once again with government officials to reach a resolution. This political subjectivity was not so much aimed at being responsible for their own individual choices in the neoliberal sense (Cruikshank 1999; Rose 1996), but rather to force government to accept responsibility for past choices that had had such devastating effects on the haemophilia population.

Mirroring government forms of calculation when preparing for action (Miller and Rose 2008 [1990]), HFNZ gathered detailed information about the membership through a national survey, finding that people had been treated differently by ACC in different regions and by different ACC officers even in the same regions. The survey performed the role of not only making people with haemophilia and hepatitis C 'visible' (as the public demonstrations did), but it also made their issues thinkable, calculable and amenable to deliberated initiatives (Miller and Rose 2008 [1990]). HFNZ used the information in their own calculations but also conveyed the general findings of the survey to the Ministry of Health in 2004.[7]

The hepatitis C subcommittee repositioned itself as a negotiating team. They decided that in their new persona as active citizens, they would act professionally, providing officials with correct information, giving credit where credit was due to Ministry officials, and criticising the Ministry on issues seen as grossly inadequate, especially in the area of treatment for hepatitis C.

Rather than claiming compensation as a citizenship right, the volunteers started to use governmental tactics of gathering technical data and collating it into policy-oriented strategy. Volunteers had long struggled to convey the complexity and urgency of the issues related to viral contamination of the blood supply. The new approach was to establish the issues as 'expert' facts, based on the survey and international best practice. They were able to show that New Zealanders were receiving poor quality treatment for hepatitis C relative to other OECD countries, and very poor quality in some regions. This act of rendering the issues 'technical' (Li 2007) meant that issues were no longer up for debate. These data were used to highlight a discourse of equity: the problem to be addressed was inequitable treatment and compensation for people who had contracted hepatitis C. They distilled the issues into just a few priorities and clear demands of government—what they called 'sound bites'. The central themes, continuously repeated, included:

- Access to best international practice treatment for hepatitis C
- An apology from Government
- Lump-sum recompense commensurate with ACC compensation
- Withdrawal of common law action

They found that sound bites were more powerful than detailed information.

Prioritisation of treatment for hepatitis C was in response to a number of members who were starting to feel major effects of the virus on their health. For them, treatment was their most urgent need. However, many still felt deeply aggrieved and expected an apology in recognition of the harm caused, so this was the second priority. In contrast to earlier campaigns, lump-sum compensation dropped to third in order of priority.

HFNZ held a National Hepatitis C Conference in April 2005. This was a significant step as people with hepatitis C came together for the first time and saw the need to respond collectively to treatment and compensation issues. HFNZ gained a better understanding of the issues facing its membership and got a mandate to advance the issues on their behalf. Another important aspect of the conference was that HFNZ invited two Irish Haemophilia Society activists so they could learn from the process used in Ireland to achieve results in relation to HIV and hepatitis C issues (Daly with Cunningham 2003; Taylor and Power 2011).

Together with knowledge gained from international networks, data were collated from the membership to make the domain they wished to influence clearly visible, knowable, and amenable to management. Their backstage interactions enabled them to be strategic when approaching front-stage encounters with government officials. Instead of putting forward a haemophilia community or interest group perspective, they used the data to profess neutrality and efficacy as they sought to mobilise government officials to address the priorities that HFNZ had identified. This strategic reversal of governmental techniques and collective action were all part of their plan to create the power to exert influence. With the issues now documented, ordered, evaluated, and made 'technical' by being based on expert rather than emotive discourse, and each issue assigned to the domain of a single spokesperson ('one person, one issue'), each spokesperson became extremely knowledgeable about 'their' issue (more knowledgeable than the people they were dealing with) and so provided brief, accurate, and consistent information: active citizenship perfected.

HFNZ's leadership's strategic approach was multidimensional and comprehensive. For example, they took a proactive approach to courting the media, which included releasing a series of fortnightly 'newsletters' to keep the issue visible in the media, and hand-delivering submissions to government to create media opportunities. They changed their long-standing practice of anonymity and agreed to provide 'the personal story' to the media, which allowed the public to see the human consequences of bureaucratic bungling and helped get the public on-side. This approach resulted in three opposition political parties committing to active support. HFNZ also demanded responses to submissions from politicians within a certain time frame. Meanwhile, it promoted self-responsibility and good citizenship in *Bloodline* articles and at education sessions by advising people how to take good care of themselves (with diet, exercise), to use treatment products wisely, and to keep careful personal health and treatment records and to make these records available to national databases. This suggested that HFNZ was a part of governmental attempts to make citizens self-regulating and responsibilised, while at the same time turning such neoliberal devices back on the state.

In early 2005, the Director General of Health, a long-time target of the HFNZ campaign and therefore knowledgeable about the issues, agreed to consider a submission from HFNZ detailing new information and a possible settlement. This was the first success of the proactive strategy. However, with the September 2005 general election fast approaching and still no agreement likely, HFNZ again reassessed their strategy, turning their attention to potential coalition parties in the next government.

Tactics of resistance: when all else fails... 2005–6

Frustrated with the drawn out 'negotiations' with the government, a member of the negotiating team pulled a stunt that brought results overnight. With just days until the parliamentary election, he created a pamphlet for a letterbox drop to all households in the Mt Albert and Rongotai electorates— seats then held by Labour members, Prime Minister Helen Clark, and Hon Annette King, the Minister of Health. King had provided the 1999 promise that she would resolve the issue with urgency if elected. The pamphlet, headed 'Labour's legacy of lies', showed a copy of King's written promise and stated:

> Labour breaks election promise. Its [sic] been six years since people with Haemophilia received a written guarantee that Labour would settle the issue of the infection of people with Haemophilia matter in a speedy and fair manner. 168 out of 171 have received no settlement offer. (HFNZ Archives)

HFNZ had learned through experience and from their Irish counterparts that the threat of public shaming was more effective than the action itself. Earlier actions undertaken to publicly shame politicians into settling the matter had been ineffective, contrary to expectations perhaps created during the pre-neoliberal era of activism in New Zealand.

Instead, the HFNZ volunteer merely approached the Minister at a public meeting and threatened to deliver the pamphlets, then waited for the response. He did not have to wait long. The next morning the negotiating team received a call from the Ministry of Health with a request for urgency in resolving the hepatitis C issue. Unbeknown to HFNZ, the Labour government had received polling information that their level of support had dropped significantly. The threatened political action could not have come at a better time (or worse time for the Labour politicians).

In the words of a key player, 'suddenly it was easy'. After 13 years of lobbying, the battle-weary volunteers suddenly managed to negotiate the terms of a settlement within two weeks. An opportunistic request for resourcing HFNZ to provide more outreach workers to support people with a bleeding disorder and hepatitis C was also agreed to by the Ministry of Health. The implementation of the settlement took considerably longer, but the haemophilia community celebrated a restored sense of justice and dignity following the agreement being reached.

In December 2006, a Treatment and Welfare package was announced, meeting HFNZ's demands. All people (not just those with haemophilia) who had contracted hepatitis C through blood or blood products were awarded equitable compensation, and provisions were made for treatment for those infected. The Prime Minister, Helen Clark, also issued a statement that acknowledged the harm done, but did not go so far as to admit fault. This statement of regret rather than apology came at a time when the New Zealand government was apologising, especially to Māori for Treaty of Waitangi transgressions. The opportunity to heal and forgive through a moral process of authentic apology (Taft 2000) was lost. People with haemophilia were left confused about why they had not received the same courtesy, and the lingering sense that they had been abandoned by the state, 'thrown on the rubbish heap', as someone had put it a decade earlier, was reinvigorated for some.

The New Zealand government was not alone in its unwillingness to admit guilt, despite the apologies offered by some other governments. The Japanese government and individual companies, for example offered a profound apology for their treatment of people with haemophilia (Schmidt 2011). In contrast, reflecting on the HIV scandal related to people with haemophilia in France and the French government's unwillingness to admit guilt, Ricoeur noted that this was an example of the increasing evidence in civil law of the concept of 'responsibility without fault' (2000, 25). This concept suggests a shift in focus away from punishing the perpetrators toward compensation for victims. This helps situate HFNZ's decision to turn their attention to achieving fair compensation and treatment for hepatitis C, rather than punishing those responsible. However, New Zealand's no-fault system existed long before this global shift toward compensatory solutions. ACC had been established to avoid litigation and provide compensation for accidents. The fact that HFNZ had spent so many years 'battling' was largely due to the inability of the existing (and new) compensation system to deal with viral contamination of the blood supply and a lack of political will to address this problem. HFNZ's demand for compensation for individuals based on a rights discourse failed, as did 'negotiation'. Despite the neoliberal political appetite for rights and responsibilities these were directed more at citizens than the state or its agents.

National restructuring of haemophilia care

Viral contaminants in the blood supply and their consequences were not the only issues that the Society was confronting during the period from 1983 to 2005. Volunteers were also lobbying to overcome regional inequalities in

Demanding Rights and Equity	Render Technical	Restructuring Governance
- Equitable access to blood products - Citizenship rights to quality standards of care	- Regional inequities in access to quality care - Develop national standards of care	- Make visible limits of regional health structure - Create national body to govern H care - Equity and inclusion discourses

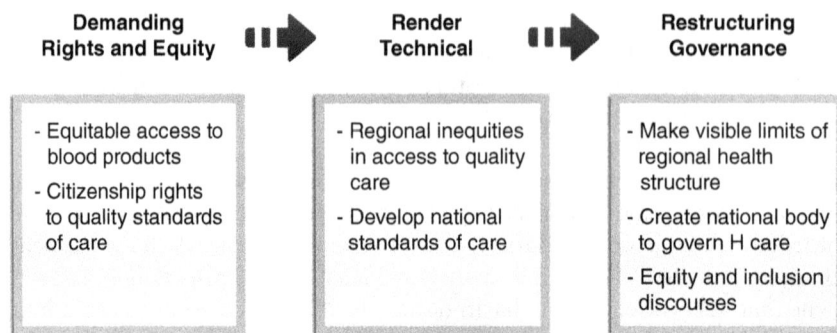

Figure 6.2 Changes in tactics to address quality of care.

access to blood products in the mid-to-late-1980s, and to address regional inequities in access to quality haemophilia care, finally achieved in 2006. Over time, volunteers developed skills, techniques, discourses, and networks that helped leverage political influence, which is why the hepatitis C story is so fundamental to understanding HFNZ's eventual success at changing the governance structure of haemophilia care. Learning from their experiences of hepatitis C, the newly formed HFNZ shifted from a demand for people's rights to quality standards of care to a demand for regional equity and inclusion in decision making (see Figure 6.2).

Because of significant chronological overlap between collective actions, we now go back in time to the 1990s to trace the emergence of HFNZ as an effective social citizen. When we began our research in 1994, inequalities in access to blood products and extremely variable standards of haemophilia care were serious concerns. While each issue had some specific peculiarities, both were largely linked to regionalisation of health services, which was at its peak at this time. For this reason, regionalised funding for blood products and haemophilia care did not work well.

Equitable access to blood products

Until 1993, blood transfusion units in New Zealand operated independently, funded by the government health budget, although there was an informal voluntary association between regions. Auckland acted as the coordinating centre and liaised on behalf of all the boards with CSL, which contracted to process New Zealand blood donations into specialised products. This system meant that there was no explicit provision for legal responsibility for the supply of blood (Howden-Chapman *et al.* 1996).

In 1993, restructuring of the health service, including the blood transfusion system, led to the six local blood transfusion units being transferred to CHEs. RHAs were to reimburse CHEs and private hospitals for the blood and blood products they used, and under the Health and Disability Act, RHAs were required to monitor the performance of purchase agreements. The supply and price were monitored by the newly established Blood Transfusion Trust, but neither the Trust nor the RHAs were responsible for the quality of the blood or blood products (Howden-Chapman *et al.* 1996).

The Haemophilia Society was deeply concerned about this highly corporatised health environment, and developed the view that a national blood service would create more equitable outcomes. They were not alone in arguing for one centralised body to oversee the collection of blood, and the manufacturing, distribution, and quality of blood products. A Ministerial Review in 1996 made this recommendation, reflecting similar recommendations by the Department of Health inquiry into hepatitis C in 1992. The 1996 review stated the establishment of a national blood service was needed to ensure national consistency of service quality, a national strategic direction for future blood service, and 'To achieve rationalisation of the service process and thereby a more efficient blood service' (NZBlood 2017). Pressure also came from clinicians, from the Haemophilia Society, and from other consumer groups such as KIDS (Kids with Immune Deficiency), who also relied on blood products. Based on our research findings of inequities in service, our research group supported this demand in a publication with another public health researcher and a haematologist (Howden-Chapman *et al.* 1996).

The argument was that concerns about inequities and safety of blood quality could be overcome if the provision of blood became the responsibility of central government through a national blood transfusion organisation. Blood should continue to be a public 'gift' and the cost of processing and supply should be met directly by central government. With a population of just 3.5 million at the time, one centralised body that could oversee the collection of blood, and the manufacturing, distribution and quality of blood products made good sense (Howden-Chapman *et al.* 1996).

This argument that a centralised system would create efficiencies contradicted the basic tenet of neoliberal reforms. Health system reforms of just three years prior were based on the opposite view that competition between regions would create greater efficiencies. Yet when a more efficient system was identified, the government moved fairly quickly to centralise the blood service, creating the national New Zealand Blood Service in 1998. This meant that purchase and supply of the plasma-derived products from the Blood Service was now nationally based. Those who oversaw this major restructuring of the blood service saw it as a matter of equity:

[By August 2000, we] had developed an integrated national service able to supply to everyone whether they were in Tairawhiti or Auckland, ensuring quality, safety and supply and positioned to meet the challenges of the future as a world class service.

(Flanagan, Mitchell, and Morland, cited in *Inform* 2003, 3)[8]

While a discourse of equity was adopted to make a case for this centralisation of the blood service, the arrangement also had considerable financial advantages. The national Blood Service was able to negotiate better processing deals than when each regional authority sourced their own products. A national body was also able to provide education about product change and associated equipment needs, and manage stockholding of treatment products, thereby eliminating problems of date-expired stock held at a regional level. The national Blood Service created processes based on a principle of 'haemovigilance' in recognition that blood and blood products are 'biologic in nature and carry inherent risks in respect of infection or reactions in the recipient' (New Zealand Blood Service 2008, 11). Following international trends, the National Haemovigilance Programme was also established in 2005, to track and monitor all activities in the blood treatment chain from blood donors to blood recipients (Mant and Smith 2013). PHARMAC, too, reportedly negotiated some of the cheapest factor VIII prices in the world (Harper 2006, 6) and took over the national purchasing of all recombinant haemophilia products.

This was all great news for the haemophilia population. While they were still far from reaching a settlement for hepatitis C at this time, they were satisfied that they had contributed to the design of national systems of blood and pharmaceutical supply. This new structure also informed their thinking on what was needed in haemophilia care.

Rights to quality haemophilia care

Equal access to quality care was a long-standing problem for the haemophilia community. Few districts had haematologists specialising in haemophilia. Haematologists had different treatment practices and there were varying procedures for accessing other necessary services. The regionalised health service, plus distance, made sharing scarce professional resources difficult. Additionally, isolation and lack of general medical expertise was a common problem for people in rural and small provincial towns (Park, Scott, and Benseman 1999).

One of the most disturbing interviews during the first phase of the research was with a young man and his family who lived in a small town in a remote part of the South Island. This teenager already had two severely damaged joints that caused him considerable pain and limited his employment options. Having met many teenagers who had no or very little joint damage, Kathryn was shocked to see that his joints looked much more like those of older men who grew up before the availability of treatment. Much of the reason for this quickly became evident. He and his family spoke about the many hours of his childhood they had spent waiting in the Accident and Emergency department of the local provincial hospital to get an infusion of blood products. In another area, he would have been whisked straight through to haematology for treatment. The young man and his mother explained that he had had many stays in hospital over his life time, reflected in the volume of his health records:

YOUNG MAN: Well, when you look at my records, they've got to bring out a trolley. [laughter]
MOTHER: They do. Oh, that day we went to theatre, and they had them stacked on his bed and two trolleys. High! 'What are these?'. 'Oh, they are his records....' I thought they were joking.

They laughed uproariously at the story, clearly not for the first time, reflecting their stoicism and ability to see the funny side of life. It also reflected a different haemophilia as a result of poor quality treatment in this remote location. Other families had moved to main centres to access good care.

Another case that also showed the lack of standardised practices was observed at a haemophilia camp. During a group discussion about treatment options, a parent explained her difficulties in getting their son treatment in a timely manner when he presented with a 'bleed' at their local hospital. In response, a haematologist from a main centre nodded and indicated that they should talk to him afterward so that he could help get a set protocol in place whereby the child would go straight to haematology. Without this chance intervention, this young child could have also progressed to debilitating joint problems.

We were told of many examples like these where some people in outlying areas experienced extremely inadequate quality of care while others reported very good care. The rarity of haemophilia meant that specialist care could not be provided everywhere. However, NZHS and HFNZ developed their view that a national system of care was necessary, demanding the right of all individuals to have equal access to quality care, including through collaboration between doctors in isolated areas and the main specialist areas of expertise. As a research participant commented in 1995, personal experiences of regional differences in standards of care helped shape this demand:

I feel quite strongly that I've experienced provincial care as well as, you know, the larger metropolitan care, the Auckland care, and they are as different as chalk and cheese ... I have a problem with that. So that's why I believe that since haemophilia seems to be quite a specialist problem or issue and because it needs such a multidisciplinary team, that we've got to change the way we are organising haemophilia care in New Zealand by having one resource centre nationally ... somewhere where the physician in Nelson or Blenheim or Oamaru is on-call, when a haemophiliac presents acutely, can ring Auckland and ask for advice. I think there's some proactive things that a resource centre could do as well, and that is issue standards of care, care protocol.

In the 1990s, a complicated mosaic of health territories was funded per head of population as described in chapter 1. The random but clustered nature of haemophilia and the high treatment costs meant that a higher than average number of people with haemophilia in a region, or a car crash involving people with haemophilia, could bankrupt a regional health service. For this reason, regionalised funding for haemophilia care did not work well. We found that throughout the country, Auckland was widely seen as the 'gold standard' in haemophilia care because of its specialist haemophilia centre. As the person quoted above exemplifies, concerns were expressed that the benefits of such a centre should not just be for those who lived in the Auckland region. This contravened the value of fairness.

National standards

The development of national standards for haemophilia care was the next step in the demand for rights to quality care. In 1993, one of the Haemophilia Society's volunteers attended the WFH Congress in Mexico and came away feeling that New Zealand was, in his words, 'Third World in terms of treatment'. He also learned that national standards of care for serious health conditions were commonplace in the UK and US at that time. This motivated him to initiate the development of similar national guidelines for New Zealand.

In 1995, the 'Standards of Care' were produced by the Haemophilia Society and its Medical Advisory Committee, in collaboration with other interested parties. In keeping with political discourses of the day, these guidelines presented a logical model of long-term financial gains and individuals' rights to best international practice. As one person explained, 'these are the sort of outcomes that we should be looking for in haemophilia care'. Governmental studies were also being undertaken to inform budgeting for future treatment (National Blood Transfusion Advisory Committee 1994; Coopers and Lybrand 1995). Financial elements of haemophilia care were clearly a priority for government.

Regionally equitable standards of care

Demanding individuals' rights to international best practice may have been a politically popular approach at the time, but, as with the viral contamination issue, a rights discourse had limited impact. Based on local and international experiences of hepatitis C and the blood service, the Society started to frame their demands in terms of equity: 'national equity' in standards of care became the new mantra.

When asked what they meant by national equity, the Society's president replied that national equity means 'ensuring that the same treatment for haemophilia care offered in large cities is offered in all areas of New Zealand' (Hardley 1997).[9] Equitable, consistent, quality care for all people with haemophilia was the goal. Hardley went on to say, 'We do not want people with haemophilia in New Zealand to be penalized for living in areas other than the main cities'. New Zealand could not support specialist haemophilia centres in all regions, but with a nationally coordinated system, NZHS determined that a more equitable and higher standard of care could be achieved. The Society also reasoned that financial savings could be achieved through a national system.

In our 2005–6 study, concerns about regional inequalities in haemophilia care standards continued. For example, a parent explained in an interview that a boy in a provincial town attended the local hospital several times before he was permitted to see the paediatrician and start treatment. Had he been in a major centre, he would have immediately been referred to a haematologist, or a paediatric haematologist if he were in Auckland. The fact that these problems continued to occur, despite greatly improved treatment options and the establishment of national guidelines, suggested that structural changes were needed to ensure greater coordination and connections between regions.

Ongoing inequities prompted the Medical Advisory Committee to develop the original Standards of Care document into the *National Guidelines— Management of Haemophilia Specification and Treatment Protocols* in 2005 (Lauzon 2008). HFNZ determined that problems related to regional inequalities in standards of care would only be overcome in the same way that regionalised blood service issues were overcome—through a nationally coordinated system of care.

With the hepatitis C settlement finally achieved in 2006, HFNZ turned its full attention to the issue of regional inequalities in haemophilia care. The volunteers worked with the Foundation's Medical Advisory Committee and government officials, using the national guidelines document to build consensus about what was needed. They were active citizens but not content to just be recognised and included in decision making. They wanted a major restructuring of haemophilia care. This type of demand is likely to be well beyond what government officials envisaged when they required local consumer involvement in planning under the New Zealand Health and Disability Act (2000).

Restructuring of national haemophilia care

In July 2006, after many years of lobbying and private conversations with government officials by HFNZ, the National Haemophilia Management Group (NHMG) was established. The NHMG includes representatives from the Haemophilia Foundation, haemophilia nurses, three haematologists, and senior officials from the Ministry of Health, the District Health Boards' (DHB's) Association, and the CEO of the New Zealand Blood Service. A national system of haemophilia care was finally created that effectively ring-fenced a national budget. DHBs now provided a population-based fee to NHMG. NHMG allocated funding for all hae-mophilia care, resulting in regional equity. In addition, NHMG worked closely with PHARMAC, which tendered for the supply of treatment prod-uct on NHMG's behalf.

HFNZ was also successful in getting two positions on the NHMG—one official and one informational. They considered their inclusion at the gov-ernance scale critical. HFNZ have found that because NHMG decisions are made by consensus, they are able to influence decisions at this level.

As a national system, the NHMG has made significant savings on treat-ment products that have been diverted, on a regionally equitable basis, to fund specialist care such as tolerisation (i.e., intensive treatment with clot-ting factors to overcome inhibitors), haemophilia nurses, physiotherapy, and elective surgery (e.g., joint replacements). All of these services make a significant contribution to quality of life and to people's ability to be involved in education, employment, and recreational activities.

An indicator of the success of the NHMG is that this national struc-ture is being replicated for other high-cost health conditions. The National Cardiac Surgery Clinical Network, for example, was established in 2009 to oversee and coordinate all cardiac surgery in New Zealand. Like the NHMG, it was also established to overcome regional inequities (Hamer and Kerr 2012). The Heart Foundation and the Cardiac Society have rep-resentation on the network but these groupings are essentially professional networks rather than voluntary patient organisations. It is difficult to deter-mine if the idea of a national structure for a costly and complex disease was translated from the haemophilia context to heart disease. Nevertheless, the same solution to regional inequities was implemented for both, thus creating a new norm of regional equity that went counter to neoliberal concepts of individual responsibility and decentralised decision making. Gauld (2012) has also outlined a trend toward post-2008 centralisation or integration of some other areas of the health system, including some of the 'back room' functions, a National Health Board and also some delivery of care initiatives, such as integrated family health centres.

Conclusion

HFNZ became a politically savvy voluntary association that is justifiably proud of the influence it has exerted over the national policies that affect its membership. As this review has revealed, during the decade between mid-1990s and mid-2000s, HFNZ attempted to assert rights of *victims* of the bad blood scandal, then to point out (but later retreat from pursuing) failures in duty of care by state agencies toward individuals, and finally promoted the responsibilities of individuals with haemophilia. This moving feast of moral imperatives closely reflected global discourses of individual rights and responsibility as they emerged and transformed throughout this period. The moral field was also shaped by expectations created through historical experiences of the haemophilia population and under existing accident compensation legislation that individuals would be compensated and perpetrators of the injury would not be punished. Changes to accident compensation laws removed these rights from many affected people with haemophilia but did not replace this loss with the right to sue the state for damages. Narratives of blame were therefore targeted at politicians who refused to reach a settlement for hepatitis C.

HFNZ was a strong voluntary association with leaders capable of harnessing global networks, well-versed in advocacy and collective action, and with expectations of partnership with clinicians and government agencies. That haemophilia is inherited and life-threatening helped create intergenerational skills, networks, and expectations to advocate collectively. The fact that HFNZ is the national organisation for all people with haemophilia (and now for other bleeding disorders), and acts independently rather than being aligned with pharmaceutical companies, enabled their volunteers to advocate at a national, central government scale.

The hepatitis C issue was finally sorted when HFNZ shifted its focus toward achieving national equity in compensation payments and quality standards of care for people affected by hepatitis C within the haemophilia community. Rather than reinscribing their marginal status by asserting their rights as victims of bad blood, as they had done in the past, they adopted an active citizen persona. This shift in subjectivity from passive to active citizen was critical as it enabled them to successfully negotiate the political field to pressure central government to make good on an earlier promise to members to reach a just settlement.

Norms of equity and inclusion were also critical in the establishment of national bodies to oversee blood supply and haemophilia care. Having asserted themselves as active citizens who were a force to be reckoned with, HFNZ went on to contribute to a national system of care.

Rather than seeking to reduce costs, HFNZ wanted to show a more innovative and equitable approach to care. Policy makers were receptive to the idea of innovation since it would not cost more and would generate better results. This was a win-win situation, where everyone wanted the same thing. As a highly knowledgeable, networked, and skilled voluntary association, HFNZ had become an extremely active citizen pursuing social citizenship goals. It was intimately involved in the design *and* ongoing implementation of a national structure. Innovation was a 'means' to restructure health structures to achieve the 'ends' of greater equity and higher standards of care.

By analysing the emergent governance structures, this chapter reveals how HFNZ mediated political, moral, and ethical forms to create new governance forms. HFNZ used its knowledge and networks created through a drawn-out period of collective action to reimagine the way haemophilia care could be governed.

They established the 'indisputable' fact that nationally equitable standards of care were the priority at this time (rather than say free physiotherapy), using scientific language, financial logic, political discourses of inclusion and equity, and global networks to influence policy. The discourse of equity proved to be effective, perhaps since the concept resonates with historical cultural preferences for a 'fair go'. Yet the new structure turns its back on decentralisation and competitive funding arrangements that are fundamental to neoliberal governmentality. We suggest that this new structure is an innovation in governance made possible by collective strategising and action by a voluntary association. Humpage (2015, 242) suggests that this kind of development is likely to become more widespread at a range of scales as national and global citizens respond to neoliberalism's challenges.

In the concluding chapter, we briefly review how, in the postsettlement phase, HFNZ was able to turn its attention to different haemophilias. It was in this period, during and after the last formal phase of our study, that moves toward a recognition of the Treaty of Waitangi within the structure and functions of HFNZ were actualised. In this period too, the different haemophilias of, for example, older men, siblings of children with haemophilia, and especially women, differently situated in the haemophilia community, could be identified and attended to. With settlement came the time, space, organisational, and emotional energy to devote to these important dimensions of different haemophilias. We also update the changing relationship between NHMG and PHARMAC. Finally we reflect on our research itself.

Notes

1. Letter from CSL Bioplasma to HFNZ, 30 August 2000. HFNZ Archives, Christchurch.
2. Not all heat treatment technologies are equally effective in inactivating HIV. Small numbers of seroconversions continued throughout the world until a collection of processes were agreed upon and implemented, and nonsafe products withdrawn (Evatt 2012).
3. In 1974, as a result of the 1973 Accident Compensation Commission, common law rights to sue for compensation for injury were replaced by fair compensation from ACC, including medical and rehabilitation, earnings-related compensation for income loss, and lump-sum payments.
4. Some examples were: NZHS letter to Hon W Birch, Minister for ACC re settlement of Hepatitis C claims, 23 June 1993; Correspondence in 1997 (7 Feb, 10 June) between NZHS and Dr Feek, MoH, re extension of recombinant product availability; meeting in November 1998; formal response from Minister of Health to NZHS 28 Jan 1999, to NZHS's 'Issues for Haemophilia In New Zealand'; correspondence in 1999, (15 and 25 Feb) re possible CKJ in Kogenate batches. HFNZ Archives, Christchurch.
5. The NZHS wrote to Minister Helen Clark in September and October 1990 with these demands. With a change in government, from Labour to National, in November 1990, Simon Upton became Minister of Health. Further letters from the Haemophilia Society, their Medical Advisory Committee, and the Regional Blood Transfusion Directors, over more than two years, were unsuccessful in getting adequate measures in place to ensure blood safety. HFNZ Archives, Christchurch.

6. Examples were: Meeting of HFNZ with Minister of Health and subsequent HFNZ letter (of 16 pages outlining the issues) to Minister re Hepatitis C Issues, 16 Dec 2000, reply of acknowledgment from Minister, 19 Dec, follow up HFNZ letter of 19 April 2001.
7. HFNZ, letter to Ministry of Health, 11 June 2004. HFNZ Archives, Christchurch.
8. *Inform* was the 'Newsletter' of the Australasian College of Health Service Management. In 2006, the College established the *Asia Pacific Journal of Health Management*. HFNZ Archives, Christchurch.
9. Peta Hardley, President, interviewed in 'Hemophilia Leader', December 1997, 4. HFNZ Archives, Christchurch

References

Biehl, J. 2005. *Vita: Life in a Zone of Social Abandonment*. Berkeley: University of California Press.

Carnahan, M.J. 2013. *Allies or Enemies: How Those Needing Help Learned to Help Themselves in the Face of Bad Blood*. Christchurch: Haemophilia Foundation of New Zealand.

Chen, S.L., and T.R. Morgan. 2006. 'The Natural History of Hepatitis C Virus (HCV) Infection'. *International Journal of Medical Sciences* 3 (2):47–52.

Coopers and Lybrand. 1995. *Prophylactic Treatment for Severe Haemophilia A: An Assessment of Costs and Benefits*. Wellington: Ministry of Health. http://www.moh.govt.nz/notebook/nbbooks.nsf/0/38ECC3AA544C56784 C256849007FC363?OpenDocument

Cruikshank, B. 1999. *The Will to Empower: Democratic Citizens and Other Subjects*. Ithaca: Cornell University Press.

Daly, R., with P. Cunningham. 2003. *A Case of Bad Blood*. Dublin: Poolbeg Press.

Davy, J. 2001 [1974]. 'John Davy'. *Bloodline* 29 (1):8.

Department of Health. 1992. 'Inquiry into Matters Relating to the Safety of Blood Products in New Zealand'. Wellington: Department of Health.

Evatt, B.L. 2012. 'The AIDS Epidemic in Haemophilia Patients II: Pursuing Absolute Viral Safety of Clotting Factor Concentrates 1985–8'. *Haemophilia* 18:649–54.

Farrell, A-M. 2006. 'Is the Gift Still Good? Examining the Politics and Regulation of Blood Safety in the European Union'. *Medical Law Review* 14 (2):155–79.

Fischer, D.H. 2012. *Fairness and Freedom: A History of Two Open Societies, New Zealand and the United States*. Oxford: Oxford University Press.

Gauld, R. 2012. 'New Zealand's Post-2008 Health System Reforms: Toward Re-centralization of Organizational Arrangements'. *Health Policy* 106 (2):110–3.

Hamer, A., and A. Kerr. 2012. 'Beyond Equity of Access to Equity of Outcome'. *New Zealand Medical Journal* 125:8–10.

Harper, P. 2006. 'Report of the HFNZ 48th Annual General Meeting, The Future of Haemophilia'. *Bloodline* (June):4–6.

Howden-Chapman, P., J. Park, K. Scott, and J. Carter. 1996. 'An Intimate Reliance: Health Reform, Viral Infections and the Safety of Blood Products'. In *Intimate Details and Vital Statistics*, edited by P. Davis, 168–84. Auckland: Auckland University Press.

Humpage, L. 2015. *Policy Change, Public Attitudes and Social Citizenship: Does Neoliberalism Matter?* Bristol: Policy Press.

Kirp, D. 1999. 'Look Back in Anger: Hemophilia and AIDS Activism in the International Tainted-Blood Crisis'. *Journal of Comparative Policy Analysis: Research and Practice* 1:177–202.

Larner, W., and D. Craig. 2005. 'After Neoliberalism? Community Activism and Local Partnerships in Aotearoa New Zealand'. In *Working the Spaces of Neoliberalism*, edited by N. Laurie and L. Bondi, 9–31. Malden, MA: Blackwell Publishing.

Lauzon, C. 2008. *Still Standing: Haemophilia Foundation of New Zealand 1958–2008*. Christchurch: Haemophilia Foundation of New Zealand Inc.

Li, T.M. 2007. *The Will to Improve: Governmentality, Development, and the Practice of Politics*. Durham: Duke University Press.

Mant, S., and M.P. Smith. 2013. 'Blood Safety'. *New Zealand Medical Journal (online)* 126 (1374):10–11.

Miller, P., and N. Rose. 2008 [1990]. 'Governing Economic Life'. In *Governing the Present: Administering Economic, Social and Personal Life*, edited by P. Miller, and N. Rose, 26–52. Cambridge, MA: Polity Press.

———. 2008 [1992]. 'Political Power Beyond the State: Problematics of Government'. In *Governing the Present*, edited by P. Miller, and N. Rose, 53–83. Cambridge, MA: Polity Press.

———. 2008 [1996]. 'The Death of the Social? Re-figuring the territory of Government,' In *Governing the Present*, edited by P. Miller, and N. Rose, 84–113. Cambridge, MA: Polity Press.

National Blood Transfusion Services Advisory Committee. 1994. 'Haemophilia: The Supply and Usage of Factor VIII'. Auckland: NBTSAC.

New Zealand Blood Service. 2008. *Transfusion Medicine Handbook 2008*. Auckland: New Zealand Blood Service. http://www.nzblood.co.nz/Clinical-information/Transfusion-medicine/Transfusion-medicine-handbook.

New Zealand Haemophilia Society. 1998. *Newsletter of NZHS*. September–October

NZBlood. 2017. 'The Creation of the New Zealand Blood Service'. https://www.nzblood.co.nz/about-nzbs/creation-of-nzbs/.

Park, J., K. Scott, J. Benseman, and E. Berry. 1995. *A Bleeding Nuisance: Living with Haemophilia in Aotearoa New Zealand*. Department of Anthropology, University of Auckland.

Park, J., K. Scott, and J. Benseman. 1999. 'Dealing with a Bleeding Nuisance: A Study of Haemophilia Care in NZ'. *New Zealand Medical Journal* 112:155–58.

Rabeharisoa, V. 2006. 'From Representation to Mediation: The Shaping of Collective Mobilization on Muscular Dystrophy in France'. *Social Science and Medicine* 62:564–76.

Resnik, S. 1999. *Blood Saga: Hemophilia, AIDS, and the Survival of a Community*. Berkeley: University of California Press.

Ricoeur, P. 2000. *The Just*. Translated by D. Pellauer. Chicago and London: The University of Chicago Press.

Rose, N. 1996. 'Governing "Advanced" Liberal Democracies'. In *Foucault and Political Reason: Liberalism, Neo-Liberalism and Rationalities of Government*, edited by A. Barry, T. Osborne, and N. Rose, 37–64. London: UCL Press.

———. 1999. *Powers of Freedom: Reframing Political Thought*. Cambridge: Cambridge University Press.

Rose, N., and C. Novas. 2005. 'Biological Citizenship'. In *Global Assemblages: Technology, Politics, and Ethics as Anthropological Problems*, edited by A. Ong and S.J. Collier, 439–63. Oxford: Blackwell Publishing.

Schmidt, P.J. 2011. 'Blood, AIDS and Bureaucracy: The Crisis and the Tragedy'. *Transfusion Medicine Reviews* 25 (4):335–43.

Shirley, I. 1990. 'New Zealand: The Advance of the New Right'. In *The Social Effects of Free Market Policies: An International Text*, edited by I. Taylor, 351–90. Hertfordshire: Harvester Wheatsheaf.

Standing, G. 2010. 'Social Protection'. In *Deconstructing Development Discourse: Buzzwords and Fuzzwords*, edited by A. Cornwall, and D. Eade, 53–67. Warwickshire: Practical Action Publishing.

Taft, L. 2000. 'Apology subverted: The Commodification of Apology'. *Yale Law Journal* 109 (5):1135.

Tasman-Jones, C. 1990. 'Hepatitis C—a Viral Disease of community Importance'. *The New Zealand Medical Journal* 103 (897):421–2.

Taylor, G., and M.P. Power. 2011. *Risk, Science and Blood: Politics, HIV, Hepatitis and Haemophilia in Ireland*. Galway: ARAN, Access to Research at NUI Galway. http://hdl.handle.net/10379/2547 (last accessed 11 Nov, 2018).

TVNZ. 1992. *Tonight* Programme. Television One. November 16.

Uvin, P. 2010. 'From the Right to Development to the Rights-Based Approach: How "Human Rights" Entered Development'. In *Deconstructing Development Discourse: Buzzwords and Fuzzwords*, edited by A. Cornwall, and D. Eade, 163–74. Warwickshire: Practical Action Publishing.

7 Conclusion

Since 1993, when this study was first mooted, much has changed—in the world of haemophilia, in anthropology, in health services, in Aotearoa New Zealand society, and in our lives, too. This chapter is devoted to overviewing past changes, to looking ahead and anticipating things to come, and to reviewing our research.

As people differently positioned in the haemophilia community, we authors have different experiences on which to draw. In the earlier chapters, we read, edited, and discussed one another's work to write our common narrative. Here, we have also done this. But we take another tack and write two narratives: one concentrating on haemophilia in Aotearoa New Zealand, the other on our research. This tactic enables us to draw on our particular backgrounds and strengths. We anticipate that the different narratives will appeal to our different imagined readers: people with haemophilia and those who care for them, academics and students in anthropology and other social sciences and health disciplines, health professionals, and members of the public interested in New Zealand society and culture, and in health.

First, we sketch in some personal details that give information on our positioning. When our project began, Julie was a new lecturer in Social Anthropology at the University of Auckland, Kathryn had just graduated with her Masters in Anthropology, Mike worked in the health sector and was a participant and advisor in the study as council member for NZHS. Deon was at school and his late mother was a parent-participant. As we complete the book, Julie is now Professor Emerita with ongoing research and writing projects in medical anthropology and New Zealand society. Kathryn completed her PhD in Anthropology in 2013 and has worked in social research and advocacy since then. Mike has retired from his position in health services, has served as President of HFNZ, continues his engagement with haemophilia services, and recently published a book on the viral contamination of the blood supply (Carnahan 2013). Deon completed his Masters of Arts in Anthropology in 2003, works in the health sector, has completed a decade as President of HFNZ, and is a member of the Board of Directors of the World Federation of Hemophilia.

In the first part of the conclusion, Mike and Deon combine to overview key changes in haemophilia in the last 70 years, and then focus particularly on recent years and current and anticipated issues relating to living with haemophilia in the twenty-first century. Mike draws on his experience as an older man with haemophilia and the various health complications that that status brings, along with his leadership positions in the haemophilia community, to reflect on changes, continuities, and hopes for the future. Mike, along with key colleagues, especially Mike Mapperson ('the two Mikes'), led and advocated for NZHS and HFNZ through the torrid times that we have described and, again with colleagues, helped achieve the settlement and welfare package and national management for haemophilia. As a person with a professional background in the health sector, he has a particular interest in health systems as they apply to haemophilia and related bleeding disorders. Deon, from a younger generation, shares this professional background with Mike as well as a history of leadership roles in national and international haemophilia organisations. He shares with Julie and Kathryn his education in Anthropology. In the second part, Kathryn and Julie, who have continued their engagement with anthropology and haemophilia over these years, consider the anthropological contribution of this research to understandings of haemophilia, to the scholarly fields of medical anthropology, and studies of Aotearoa New Zealand society.

Deon and Mike: change and cycles in living with haemophilia

Since World War II, people with haemophilia in New Zealand have had a range of issues dominate their lives. Seventy-odd years ago, the need was for scientific diagnosis, rather than relying on observation and family trees; then it was elementary treatment to prevent death. The decades of the 1960s and 1970s brought what are now the early fractionated blood products. Next was the golden period of these products fractionated from human plasma. This era also introduced us to blood-borne diseases, resulting in the focus turning to solving the ravages of HIV. This was followed by more disease—the hepatitis alphabet, notably hepatitis C, and the scare of variant Creutzfeldt-Jakob disease—all from blood-based plasmas. The transmission of disease by human blood brought greater demand for manufactured, nonblood-based, products. Manufactured recombinant products also became the key to improving care and assisted the extension of prophylaxis. This improved dramatically the health status of people with target joints and muscles damaged by bleeding in earlier life, and formed a solid foundation for newborns to grow without recurrent and damaging childhood bleeds. Access to manufactured products also assisted the introduction of managed care using a comprehensive care model, both at the national planning level of the National Haemophilia Management Group (NHMG), and also at the point of service delivery to individuals, with haematologist, physiotherapist, nurse specialist, dentist, social worker, and sometimes other specialists, notably in orthopaedics, cooperating to improve the individual's state of health.

During the 1990s and beyond, advocacy became the major issue in an effort to change the way treatment was organised and delivered. There were also the continuing issues of overcoming disease and improving access to manufactured products, which allowed the advent of haemophilia surgery, often involving joint replacement. Various manufactured products also permitted advances in tolerisation to achieve clotting in those who had developed antibodies to plasma-derived or recombinant products. Advocacy was also needed as new organisations appeared within health, such as PHARMAC and ACC. The introduction of PHARMAC to undertake the role of national purchaser not only brought a uniform price but also greater surety of supply and access to alternative products, plus stability, as contracts were for supply over multiple years. There would also be unintended consequences, realised later, of the formation of this national purchaser. This was also the era of a new focus on ethical issues, particularly in genetics, but also in the use of treatment products. Revisions to governmental policy, health reforms, changes to funding models, advances in science, increased genetic testing, shifting population demographics, changes to treatment protocols, and revised definitions or categorisations of bleeding, to name a few, impacted our community. What it means to live with a bleeding disorder in New Zealand, and indeed all over the world, has changed. The 'reality' of both the diagnosis and prognosis of haemophilia, other bleeding disorders, rare clotting factor deficiencies, and carrier status is dynamic.

What does it mean now to live with a bleeding disorder in Aotearoa New Zealand?

A family who would have once been introduced to a society to assist haemophiliacs (a term long out of the official community vernacular), now finds an organisation for people with bleeding disorders. A child once condemned to not live past 20 years of age can now expect to have a near-normal life expectancy. For many, bleeds are elusive with the advent of prophylaxis. Some individuals can go for many years before experiencing that 'tingling feeling' in a joint; a telltale indication of a bleed. Options for genetic testing are ever-expanding, and create some challenging ethical considerations for our community. So too does the question of how much product we should use, given its cost, and other demands on the health dollar.

Living with a bleeding disorder now should mean access to comprehensive care, a concept that goes beyond treatment with factor replacement alone. Indeed, each person with haemophilia is required to have at least one review each year. Access to adequate factor replacement therapy is pivotal, but this does not diminish the importance of access to haematologists continuing to specialise in haemophilia, physiotherapists, nurse specialists, treatment centres, dental care, and psychosocial support. After more than a decade of the NHMG in New Zealand, the majority receive this comprehensive model that has proven its value for both the people it serves, and the fiscal constraints it is subject to. The contrast between younger members of the same community experiencing no bleeds whatsoever, to elders' daily chronic pain emphasises the significant advances in treatment and the huge advantage of adequate, continuing treatment. One of Mike's young relatives, for example, 'with severe factor IX, aged nine years, has no target joints, no portacath, no time off school, and has had one trip to hospital in his lifetime'. This is a typical portrait for the younger generation.

Towards the future

To leave it there would be to oversimplify the work ahead for HFNZ. Subtle changes to policy have led to some erosion of the NHMG model. In themselves, they are minor. Taken together, these changes have the potential to move away from a world-leading model that has redirected the savings realised by PHARMAC's tender process directly back into care for people with bleeding disorders. As people with bleeding disorders are in it for the long-term, foreseeing unintended consequences of policy decisions is a particular strength of this community. The ability to plan, manage, and carry out treatments such as tolerisation or plan joint replacement surgeries, for example, is an important function of the NHMG. With more resources being directed away from the NHMG to PHARMAC's 'Combined pharmaceutical budget' (see Box 7.1), savings realised have the potential to be lost in a sea of funding decisions. HFNZ continues in its role in advocacy and bridging gaps in institutional memory due to the continuing churn in the relevant health bureaucracies with which it deals. In doing so, it insists on its hard-won expertise, its long view, and on comprehensive, nationally equitable, care for haemophilia.

In extracts from a 2013 letter to the incoming chair of the NHMG (see Box 7.1 below), HFNZ explains the purpose of the NHMG and how the proposal from PHARMAC for an organisational change cannot fulfil all the NHMG goals. Despite all the past struggles and successes, maintaining optimal systems requires constant work and constant vigilance. Successful systems face constant erosion. In this story, HFNZ is the stayer with the long-term wisdom; health systems and their personnel come and go as does institutional knowledge. The formal networks of care are unstable. This means that gains and improvements have to be regained on a cyclical basis with the ebb and flow of the people and organisations that make up the health system.

An important point that this letter conveys is that haemophilia treatment is not just a matter of clotting factor replacement, although adequate clotting factor replacement is crucial. In no group of people with haemophilia

Box 7.1

Extracts from a letter on 8 August 2013 from the CEO of HFNZ to the incoming chair of the NHMG (with permission of HFNZ)

The Haemophilia Foundation of New Zealand (HFNZ) wishes to raise some items concerning PHARMAC's letter proposing to include the management of recombinant factor products as part of their responsibility of managing hospital pharmaceuticals and medical devices. It is the hope of HFNZ that this is indeed still in the proposal stage as we believe that there are implicit risks in adopting this model without careful consideration. It appears that PHARMAC's proposal could diminish the ability of the National Haemophilia Management Group (NHMG) to continue with comprehensive national oversight despite the assertion that no change is proposed to the arrangements that are in place in relation to the role of the NHMG or the Treaters' Group [i.e., haemophilia specialists].

Given the hereditary and life-long nature of haemophilia and related bleeding disorders, our members have been recipients of many iterations of health service provision in New Zealand. We are therefore well positioned to offer a long-term view as to the risks and benefits of various models utilised. The establishment of the NHMG has been one of the most valuable developments for all people affected by haemophilia and related bleeding disorders in terms of improving both the quality of, and access to, care in New Zealand. It is therefore imperative that any new proposals do not diminish or undermine the current governance structure of the NHMG and do not put the current "ring-fenced" funding allocation at future risk. Any decisions made now will continue to affect our members well into the future.

The letter from PHARMAC implies that this agency has not been fully briefed about the background, structure and rationale of haemophilia management in New Zealand. As part of any on-going dialogue with PHARMAC, it will remain important for the NHMG to serve as an adviser in this regard. ... It is important that this earlier context is not lost. ...

The NHMG was set up to provide national consistency in access to care for all people with haemophilia and related bleeding disorders in a financially sustainable way. The two primary aims of PHARMAC's widened role are providing national consistency in access to hospital medicines and devices and creating efficiencies in spending. The parallels of the two bodies are evident. HFNZ believes that the infrastructure of consistent, high-quality haemophilia care combined with sound financial management exist under the current [NHMG] model.

The role of the NHMG is not limited to simply supplying factor replacement therapies and has included the funding of salaries for haemophilia nurses in the haemophilia treatment centres and physiotherapists in some, but not all, centres. There is no clarity in the proposed alterations as to how these positions will continue to be funded....

DHBs currently do not fund haemophilia care to appropriate levels. This has made it necessary for the NHMG to step in and fund some nursing and physiotherapy ... [staff positions]. This has resulted in improved outcomes for patients and associated cost savings. While PHARMAC already has a central role in the procurement and funding of haemophilia products, shifting the bulk of the haemophilia budget to a combined pharmaceutical budget potentially opens up a range of risks for the haemophilia patient that the NHMG are currently able to contain. ....

Recombinant factor products are presently defined as hospital pharmaceuticals. These products are predominantly consumed by patients in the community whose contact with healthcare facilities is minimal. The NHMG is the only group that has oversight of patients by way of review, and the management of their consumption of products. It is therefore implicit that to adequately treat these people, the NHMG must be the custodian of all funds allocated for haemophilia care in NZ. In believing the NHMG must control all the funds allocated for haemophilia, HFNZ also believe PHARMAC must continue to undertake national procurement. The NHMG should determine the annual needs for recombinant products; with the funding of purchases taking place at the point of procurement as has been the practice since 2006. ...

is this more evident than among the elders, due to the results of inadequate treatment in their youth. Aging and haemophilia were once words not seen in the same sentence. With life expectancy of people with haemophilia rising, the associated complications of older age are having an impact on our community. The need for multiple medications, care, and health promotion to mitigate the increased risk of falls, the effects of living with HIV and hepatitis C for decades, and the many other potential comorbidities of aging all add to the challenges of living a long, full life with a bleeding disorder.

With adequate treatment for young people, success in clearing hepatitis C, and effective tolerisation for those with inhibitors, in future, the group likely to have the greatest health demands are middle-aged to older persons living with haemophilia. Born before lab-based diagnosis, treatment, or adequate treatment, this is a group with multiple needs. Although most have few bleeds compared with their younger years, many have multiple target joints and have had, sometimes repeated, joint replacements. Their veins may be 'shot' because of treatments. Some have lost their partners and other age mates, and, in addition to haemophilia and its complications, some have developed nonhaemophilia-related conditions. This group requires complex, coordinated health resources, and will continue to do so for the next 20 or so years. Consequently, the need for expertise around the NHMG table, and amongst treating clinicians, is no longer solely in therapeutic products but also in corrective surgery and the other health issues created by this new phenomenon of aging with haemophilia. A national group is essential to plan for these and unknown future needs to optimise living with haemophilia into old age. The NHMG may need to change its skills from time to time with changing challenges. Yet, one constant that requires continuing vigilance as organisational and personnel changes occur is ensuring that a national standard of care is always in place and is adequately delivered in all the centres that treat haemophilia across Aotearoa New Zealand.

In the immediate future, factor replacement therapy is on the verge of another step-change. Extended half-life factor VIII and factor IX is a reality already for parts of the United States and some members of the European Union. As part of the World Federation of Hemophilia's Humanitarian Aid Programme, longer half-life products are being donated to many emerging economies. This therapy received United States Food and Drug Administration approval in 2014 and, in May 2016, longer-acting factor IX was approved by the European Commission. Subject to PHARMAC's next tender round, access to these products in New Zealand should be imminent. The impact of this new technology is particularly significant for older people, as a reduction in the number of needles required per week is profound in its effect of preserving veins. Mike comments, 'I'm anxiously awaiting access to long life factor IX therapy so as to ease the pressure on exhausted veins'.

These changes in technology now signal the community grappling with a new vocabulary that includes pegylation, binding immunoglobulin protein, an anti-inflammatory treatment, and genetic fusion with albumin to extend factor half-life. These terms are loaded with meaning for a community presented with the likelihood of factor replacement therapy that improves quality of life. With these technologies and the proliferation of copies of other products, the smorgasbord of treatment options promises much. However, what will be delivered in New Zealand will depend on the always-needed voice of the Foundation working with the many decision makers. On the horizon is the development of a 'tissue factor pathway inhibitor' (a protein crucial to the clotting process), which in reality means the potentiality of taking a pill for the treatment of haemophilia. New Zealanders continue to volunteer for gene therapy trials when international trials are offered.

Longer-acting therapies form part of the picture of a major step-change. Trials for gene therapy are showing promise, with individuals on trials sustaining factor levels following therapy and effectively being 'cured' of haemophilia. This therapy is mooted as becoming available for adult populations, as its success amongst children is not established. While there is some way to go in validating the efficacy of gene therapy, other questions already emerge: the cost, who will have access, and how will it impact on the treatment model for bleeding disorders? Gene therapy is not within the purview of haematology.

Even without these future hopes, the changes in understanding how to manage bleeding disorders continue to fuel debates on treatment best practice. What should trough levels of factor really be? How much factor replacement should be used to maintain appropriate levels? Who defines 'appropriate'? These debates continue to highlight how the economic reality of the cost of these therapies restricts delivering the best possible care. The savings made by using less-than-adequate factor replacement therapy now would more than likely tax the health system in years to come through the extra services required by older people with joint problems. Despite knowing the human cost of overly conservative treatment over many decades, it is typical of many haemophilia community members to continue to have a conservative approach to treatment.

Our community does not need to look far to understand how short-term savings can lead to long-term cost. The savings realised by delaying the heat treatment of factor therapies to remove hepatitis C have been spent many times over by the resultant need to treat those New Zealanders who received contaminated blood and blood products. This early decision did not affect all people living with hepatitis C, but it does account for many people in our community who have lived or continue to live with or have successfully cleared the virus. With new therapy for hepatitis C funded through ACC for our community and the flow-on to the wider community with funding through PHARMAC, ultimately, living hepatitis C-free is a reality for the majority of people with the virus. The long-term benefits will be profound.

Mike was one of those who had to wait for the new generation of anti-hepatitis C drugs to clear it, despite several earlier attempts. He writes, 'Since 2013 I have "done Sofosbivir" [a new anti-hepatitis C drug] as part of a trial and managed to clear HCV, along with the other 15 people with haemophilia who did the trial at the time I did. I also agreed to participate in the following three-year monitoring programme which finished Nov 2016'. Deon, in contrast, went through the 'old' hepatitis C treatment in the early 2000s and for him it was successful, but he comments that 'this was not the reality for many who went through the earlier generation treatment'. Hepatitis C treatment has become much more effective over time.

By 2016, the definition of the group of New Zealanders with bleeding disorders expanded to include women as people with, as well as carriers of, haemophilia—although HFNZ acknowledged this much earlier. People with other bleeding disorders, such as those with von Willebrand disease and those with rare factor deficiencies, are also members and represented by HFNZ. It is now widely acknowledged that even among women who may have relatively high factor levels, 'microbleeds' can still occur leading to joint damage. With such definitional changes, language has shifted to refer to everyone as living with a bleeding disorder.

Within the haemophilia and other bleeding disorders community, recognition of the Treaty of Waitangi and specifically Māori issues has been enacted in the formation of Piritoto, one of the formal groups within HFNZ that has representation on Council. The needs of young people, women, older people, and members of the diverse ethnicities which constitute the diversifying population of Aotearoa New Zealand and the haemophilia community, are recognised through specific groups, networks, activities, and programmes.

What are the challenges for haemophilia in New Zealand over the next 20 years? In summary, the greatest medical issue will be dependence on and access to therapeutic products should gene therapy either not deliver as expected, or not be made available. Anything that might upset access to therapeutic products—whether it be presence in the products of something injurious to health, upset to supply such as a natural or human-made disaster, or problems of interruption to temporary or long-term supply, such as legislative restriction, or New Zealand's inability or reluctance to pay for supplies—would be catastrophic. Similarly, should gene therapy prove safe and effective, delaying access could arguably mirror earlier decisions made for short-term cost savings that had longer-term cost implications. Within the health sector, the maintenance of an equitable system delivering haemophilia care of a high and uniform standard across the country will continue to be crucial in ensuring that all New Zealanders can benefit. Complementing this is a need to be aware of and respond to the most vulnerable groups of people living with haemophilia. For the near future, this will include the elderly.

A continuing challenge is the enduring social need for people with bleeding disorders to get together, support each other, and offer a community of understanding. A group that began by supporting people with severe haemophilia now covers the whole range of bleeding disorders and the changing demographic profile of the haemophilia community reflects the changes in New Zealand society over time. Ensuring voice and recognition within the wider community, along with personal support and advocacy remain crucial. So too does the voice and advocacy of HFNZ on the national and international scene, respectful of the fact that we are one organisation among many sharing the common resources of citizens.

Kathryn and Julie: different haemophilia and local biology in Aotearoa New Zealand

At the beginning of our book, we explained that we wanted to make an up-close account of what it is like to live in Aotearoa New Zealand with a condition in which blood takes too long to clot. We argued that although haemophilia is well understood in medical and genetic terms as a result of mutations in one of two genes located on the X chromosome, even in a single nation with a common public health system, the experience of this condition is multiple. Despite this diversity, the shared social and cultural conditions of Aotearoa New Zealand produce what we can call a local biology of haemophilia. This everyday, lived experience of haemophilia in Aotearoa New Zealand, which we explore as a multidimensional cultural phenomenon, is the focus of this book. We offer it as a complement to more medically or psychologically focussed research and to studies located in other nations.

We hope that readers within the international haemophilia community, and other biosocial communities formed around comparable conditions, will identify commonalities and differences of experience when comparing their own lives and communities with those of people in Aotearoa New Zealand. Despite the global commonalities, local history, culture, politics and economics will continue to shape people's experiences and choices. For a nation the size of New Zealand with an estimated population of 4.76 million in 2018, having a centralised system of haemophilia governance, a national blood and pharmaceutical service, and a single patient advocacy group has demonstrable advantages. Is this model transposable to other jurisdictions, and is it relevant to other rare conditions? We think so, and hope that health systems scholars, practitioners, and community members will engage with these ideas. Another transposable lesson is that of having courage and persistence to collectively challenge systems that seem set in stone, whether they be gender structures or health systems. Our research findings and the New Zealand haemophilia community itself, for example, have been part of a global shift away from men 'having haemophilia' and women 'carrying haemophilia' and of health system change.

Different haemophilia and local biology

We have followed our ethnographic noses to investigate what matters most to people with haemophilia, their families, and health professionals. This has led us to write in detail about experiences like the traumas of learning that your child has haemophilia, learning to give home treatments on their tender and wriggling little bodies, the sadness of 'not rugby', the issues of hepatitis C, the moral dilemmas of being part of changing technologies and networks of care, and political struggles for national haemophilia management. These ethnographic narratives of Aotearoa New Zealand are situated in wider contexts, in relation to gender, social policy, new technologies, and in relation to a range of useful anthropological theory, as we attempt to combine the immediacy of the personal and local with the broader issues with which they engage. Anthropology is well-recognised for its gift of ethnography to understanding and writing about social life; just as important is its contribution to the theoretical tool kit with which we seek to systematically and critically think through the complexities of social life (Fitzgerald and Park 2003).

The multiplicity of the experience of haemophilia is one of our key themes. The biology of haemophilia, which creates difference through severity, type, and ability to respond to treatment, creates a level of complexity. Interwoven with this are personal characteristics such as when you were born, whether you are male or female, where you live, your family history, and social context, to make these differences further complex. Personal and family narratives about haemophilia, which give value to life and experience, also mediate people's meanings and experiences of haemophilia. Whether one is a person with haemophilia, a family member, a medical caregiver, or a scientist is key to creating different haemophilias. These personal differences interact in complex ways with broader socio-historical dimensions including social arrangements, cultural values, social provision, organisation of the health system, economic conditions, networks of technology, government policy, and community organisations. It is these multilevel interactions that produce different bodily experiences and understandings of haemophilia: why for one person it is 'just a bleeding nuisance', while for another it is to be avoided at all costs.

When we talked to people living with haemophilia, much of their talk was not so much about dealing with the bodily effects of haemophilia, but more about how it shaped their experiences and aspirations in their daily life—their education, relationships, leisure activities, and employment—and their senses of self. We show the implications for many aspects of life from infancy to old age. These different haemophilias do have commonalities that create local biologies of haemophilia. National narratives in which cultural values are entailed are part of the experience. When we began our study of living with haemophilia, we did not anticipate that a few of the things for which New Zealand is internationally well-known—rugby, and the New Right neoliberal 'experiment'—would turn out to be so important in the haemophilia community. These are examples of how global shifts, local restructures, and cultural norms coalesce to create local biologies of haemophilia: another of our key themes.

Local biologies are especially visible when making international comparisons, or comparing haemophilia over time. For example, people with haemophilia in New Zealand can now expect to be adequately treated at little personal financial cost and can expect to have an average life expectancy. A sense of inclusive citizenship also works within this biosocial community so that an ethic of conserving expensive national health resources is evident, although not universal. The national rates of blood-borne infections in the past can be compared internationally and explained by the way technological networks, including blood bank and fractionation services, were organised, and the background population infection rates and political responses. The relatively low uptake of prenatal testing can be related to local views of the seriousness of haemophilia, the worth of lives with haemophilia, and cultural values about having biological children, as well as how genetic services are organised and funded. How national haemophilia services are currently organised can be traced to aspects of national politics, recourse to the value of 'a fair go', the specific history of HFNZ, its close relationship with its medical advisors, and changing relationships with government.

One of the advantages of the size of Aotearoa New Zealand is that a national study of a rare condition is entirely feasible. Consequently, this national scale, long-term study of living with haemophilia is a unique contribution to health and haemophilia studies and medical anthropology. We have been able to consider how the specific ways in which Aotearoa New Zealand society is gendered contribute to the local biology of haemophilia and how that is changing. We were privileged to delve into the moral decision-making of men and women especially around testing girls for having a haemophilia gene and about prenatal testing. We concluded that, although such tests are medically routine, they are far from routine for people with haemophilia. Our work has detailed how ongoing health reforms, new technologies, and viral contamination coalesce to create specific expectations and experiences. Experience with genetically modified treatment products, we suggest, makes people with haemophilia more open to gene therapy than their location in 'GE free' New Zealand might indicate. These specific aspects of the local biology of haemophilia lead us to endorse the value of researching at the national level, and of working with deeply considered 'lay' understandings of genetics, eugenics, and the value of life (Franklin and Roberts 2006, 222).

Throughout the preceding chapters, we have shown how the ever-changing health structures over several decades are linked to global and local political shifts and how they directly impact people's lives, including at the most basic level: being able to walk unaided or knowing you will be cared for if you become really sick. These ethnographic accounts make the consequences of changing organisational technologies visible and graspable at the personal and family level. These technologies are embodied by people with haemophilia.

We revealed that members of the haemophilia community take a measured approach to new technologies, aware of their history, with people willing to look for the benefits as well as the possible disadvantages when considering their adoption. The community has developed an approach to the inevitable differences of opinion and values that emerge as part of new technologies; an approach that combines choice, caring, and the public withholding of moral judgement, expressed in the commonly heard phrase: 'What's right for the family is what's right'. In this regard, the past and present provide clues about the new networks of care that are sure to arise in the future.

Studying haemophilia/studying Aotearoa New Zealand

While this has indeed been an account of the experience of haemophilia in a specific national context, as the concepts of local biologies and different haemophilias suggest, it is simultaneously a broader study of Aotearoa New Zealand society and changes in this society over the last few decades. New Zealand is known as one of the most rapidly neoliberalising nations, but our research shows that this is not a wholesale transformation in values or practices. The sediments of welfare state values of social participation, care, and reciprocity are not sealed in neat strata completely covered with a thick stratum of neoliberalism with its values of choice, freedom, and active citizenship. Rather, as perhaps suitable in these earthquake-prone and volcanic shaky isles, there is a rich and often confusing folding and fracturing of strata, making sometimes contradictory values available as rhetorical and interpretative resources for citizens and government. HFNZ, for example, was eventually able to use the practices of active citizenship and a rhetoric of equity to achieve its goal of a government treatment and welfare package in response to hepatitis C and its goal of a national system of management of haemophilia. However, it was not successful in gaining a full apology. Instead, it received an expression of regret: care but no responsibility. Our theorising of the personal and community experiences of the blood-borne viruses and the associated government response as social suffering provides an example of the effects of this suffering not just on the individuals, families, and community but on the political system and ultimately the health care system for people with haemophilia and therefore on haemophilia itself.

The study contributes to knowledge of social citizenship in New Zealand (Humpage 2015). We show that members of the haemophilia community are cognisant of the costs to society of their treatment as well as the personal and social costs of nontreatment. In this neoliberalised nation, the haemophilia community demonstrates a sense of national citizenship: that all citizens are entitled to a fair go and to have health care that promotes a 'normal life', however that might be understood. At the same time, given scarce resources, an often-noted value is that everyone needs to be aware—and some would urge, careful of—the demands made on health and other services so that there are sufficient resources for others. Practical expression of this value by people with haemophilia might be as routine as being careful of expiry dates for treatment products, as difficult as not playing rugby, or as intimate and momentous as decisions about family size or using prenatal technologies. Perhaps this is one part neoliberal responsibilisation, one part social welfare-ist social participation, and one part an older ideal of moderation and fairness.

References

Carnahan, M.J. 2013. *Allies or Enemies: How Those Needing Help Learned to Help Themselves in the Face of Bad Blood*. Christchurch: HFNZ.

Fitzgerald, R., and J. Park. 2003. 'Introduction: Issues in the Practice of Medical Anthropology in the Antipodes'. *Sites (NS) Medical Anthropology: Tales from the Antipodes* 1 (1):1–29.

Franklin S., and C. Roberts. 2006. *Born and Made: An Ethnography of Pre-Implantation Genetic Diagnosis*. Princeton: Princeton University Press.

Humpage, L. 2015. *Policy Change, Public Attitudes and Social Citizenship: Does Neoliberalism Matter?* Bristol: Policy Press.

Glossary

amniocentesis   A prenatal test on amniotic fluid to detect a chromosomal abnormality

a fair go   A colloquial protest or plea for more fairness or reason

antibodies   Protective immunoglobulin protein produced by the immune system in response to the presence of a foreign substance (or antigen). Antibodies recognise and latch onto antigens to remove them from the body.

antibody tests   An analysis (usually of blood) to determine the presence or amount of antibody.

arthropathy   Disease of the joints

calliper   A splint made of metal rods and leather (or similar) straps designed to support and or exert tension on the leg.

carrier   A woman who carries a haemophilia mutation gene. About 30 per cent of women carriers have lower clotting factor levels. Three times more women carry these mutations than do men.

cirrhosis of the liver   Scarring and loss of liver cells

'clean green' image   An image represented by snow-capped mountains, clean air, and rivers with pristine green fields.

clotting factors   Proteins in the blood that control bleeding and clotting

Crown   A complex symbol. It may refer to the monarchy, the government, parliament, or the State.

Creutzfeldt-Jakob disease   A degenerative brain disease caused by abnormal prion proteins

epigenetic phenomena   Alternative states of gene expression

fractionation   The process of separating the components of blood plasma. A step in the production of clotting factor replacement treatments.

gene therapy   The insertion of a desired gene into a cell to replace a defective gene —in the case of haemophilia, to stimulate clotting factor production.

getting the run around   Intentional unclear, misleading, incomplete, or evasive information, especially in a response to a question or request.

Haemophilia (UK) Hemophilia (US)   An X chromosome genetic condition where specific clotting factors are absent or at lower than normal levels so that blood is slow to clot resulting in prolonged bleeding or oozing after an injury or surgery. In severe cases, heavy bleeding occurs after minor injury or may occur spontaneously.

haemophilia A   In the clotting cascade, factor VIII is missing or low, resulting in clotting becoming disrupted.

haemophilia B   In the clotting cascade, factor IX is missing or low, resulting in clotting becoming disrupted.

haka   Chant/dance of challenge and/or greeting; shows respect

hepatitis   Any inflammation of the liver. Hepatitis B and C are caused by viruses and have infected people with haemophilia through treatment products

hepatitis: non-A non-B   Hepatitis caused by any number of infectious agents not detectable by methods that reveal the presence of hepatitis A and B.

hepatitis A   Infectious hepatitis, marked by an incubation period of 1–3 weeks, faecal-oral transmission, a high degree of contagiousness; an acute self-limited illness, possibly protracted and severe (even fatal) but does not result in chronic hepatitis or cirrhosis.

hepatitis B/serum hepatitis   Serum hepatitis, or hepatitis B, marked by a longer incubation period of 1–3 months, parenteral or sexual transmission, a low degree of contagiousness; an acute illness, usually self-limited but can be severe or fatal and also result in chronic infection, chronic hepatitis and even cirrhosis.

hepatitis C or hep C   A blood-borne virus causing inflammation of the liver marked by slow onset and nonspecific symptoms ranging from relatively mild to extensive cirrhosis, liver failure or liver cancer.

hepatitis C test   A blood test that identifies the genetic material (RNA) of the virus or antibodies (proteins) that the body makes against it

home treatment   Intravenous infusion of replacement clotting factor carried out by the person with haemophilia or a household member

half-life of factor   The time taken for the activity level of replacement clotting factor in the blood to drop to 50 per cent

inhibitors   Antibodies that destroy replacement clotting factor

interferon   Proteins produced in the body that assist immune response. Interferon is used in treatments, e.g., for hepatitis C, and gives rise to flu-like symptoms

iwi   Tribe, bone, people

karyotyping   Analysis of chromosomes to detect abnormalities

liver function test   Commonly used tests to check liver function. E.g., the alanine transaminase (ALT), aspartate aminotransferase (AST), alkaline phosphatase (ALP), albumin, and bilirubin tests. The ALT and AST tests measure enzymes that the liver releases in response to damage or disease.

locum   A temporary replacement often for a medical specialist

Māori   The indigenous people of Aotearoa New Zealand

marae   Māori ceremonial and community centre

Mirena® iud   An interuterine device that releases a hormone that assists some women who have menstrual difficulties

obligate carrier   All daughters of men with haemophilia have the same mutation as their father.

on-demand treatment   Treatment administered after a bleed has started

outreach workers   Staff of HFNZ who support families with haemophilia

Pākehā   The settler-derived population of New Zealand. It is a contested term.

pegylation   The modification of biological molecules by attachment or amalgamation of polyethylene glycol polymer chains to give targeted drug therapy

pegylated interferon   Viral eradication using antiviral therapy based on the use of a combination of three different drugs

pegylated ribavirin   An early antiviral medication

Piritoto   The Māori group within Haemophilia Foundation of New Zealand (Inc) that has representation on its National Council

Plunket   The national well-child organisation

political football   An issue that is seized on by opposing political parties

pooled plasma   Collection of human blood plasma from numerous donors for manufacture of various blood derivatives such as clotting factors

polio   A viral disease that results in muscle wasting

portacath   A device that is surgically inserted, usually in the chest, to provide venous access

privatisation   The transfer of a business, industry, or service from public to private ownership and control, usually on the grounds of improved efficiency or the need for further investment

prophylactic treatment   Clotting factor replacement treatment given on a regular basis to raise the trough or low point of clotting factor levels

recombinant products   Often written rFVIII or rFIX; synthetic clotting factor produced by PCR

Rogernomics   Neoliberal economic policies to reduce the size and role of the State, followed by Roger Douglas as Minister of Finance in the Fourth Labour Government of New Zealand from 1984.

rugby   Often regarded as Aotearoa's national game, rugby is a contact sport played with an oval ball, played in NZ from 1870s, originally by men only

severity of haemophilia   Usually classified as severe (less than 1% of normal clotting factor levels), moderate (1% up to 5%), mild (5% to 40%)

spontaneous bleeding   Bleeding for which there is no external cause

sporadic haemophilia   Haemophilia that is the result of a recent mutation. It will be inherited in the usual way.

Starship   National children's hospital located in Auckland

surrogate testing   Testing for something commonly associated with the problem in question, such as hepatitis B, before there was a test for hepatitis C

tangata whenua   People of the land – Māori; first people of Aotearoa

target joint   A joint into which there have been repeated bleeds

tolerisation   Treatment to try and overcome inhibitors, usually given to youngsters. It uses large amounts of treatment products.

treatment (for haemophilia)   The infusion of clotting factor replacement

Treaty of Waitangi   Founding document of Aotearoa New Zealand signed in 1840 at Waitangi, and then in other places, between representatives of Queen Victoria and many Māori chiefs

trough levels   Part of the drug monitoring protocol, being the lowest concentration reached by a drug before the next dose

tūrangawaewae   'A place to stand'; home; district to which one has strong kinship ties

viral inactivation   Rendering a virus unable to infect, e.g., via solvent/detergent and heat

von Willebrand disease   A coagulation disorder that affects the von Willebrand factor

Index

For Product Safety Concerns and Information please contact our EU
representative GPSR@taylorandfrancis.com
Taylor & Francis Verlag GmbH, Kaufingerstraße 24, 80331 München, Germany

www.ingramcontent.com/pod-product-compliance
Lightning Source LLC
Chambersburg PA
CBHW060406220326
41598CB00023B/3033